The Physiology of the Joints

To my Wife

The Physiology of the Joints

Annotated diagrams of the mechanics of the human joints

I. A. Kapandji

Ancien Interne des Hôpitaux de Paris
Ancien Chef de Clinique—Assistant des Hôpitaux de Paris
Membre de la Société Française d'Orthopédie et de Traumatologie
Membre de la Société Française de Chirurgie de la Main

Translated by
L. H. HONORÉ   BSc MB CHB FRCP(C)

Foreword by
The late PROFESSOR G. CORDIER
Former Dean of the Faculty of Medicine of Paris

FIFTH EDITION

Volume 2
Lower Limb

1. The Hip
2. The Knee
3. The Ankle
4. The Foot
5. The Plantar Vault

With 690 illustrations by the author

CHURCHILL LIVINGSTONE
EDINBURGH LONDON MELBOURNE AND NEW YORK 1987

CHURCHILL LIVINGSTONE
An imprint of Elsevier Science Limited

English edition of the Second Edition 1970
English edition of the Fifth Edition 1987
  Reprinted 1989, 1991, 1994, 1995 (twice), 1998, 2001, 2002

The original French edition is entitled *Physiologie Articulaire* and
is published by Librairie Maloine, Paris

ISBN 0 443 03618 7

British Library Cataloging in Publication Data
Kapandji, I. A.
    The physiology of the joints: annotated
    diagrams of the mechanics of the human
    joints. -5th ed.
    Vol. 2: Lower limb...
    1. Joints
    I. Title   II. Physiologie articulaire.
    English
    612'.75   QP303

1003593793 ↑

Library of Congress Cataloging in Publication Data
Kapandji, I. A. (Ibrahim Adalbert)
    The physiology of the joints.

    Translation of: Physiologie articulaire.
    Includes bibliographies.
    Contents: - v. 2. Lower limb.
    1. Human mechanics. 2. Joints - Atlases. I. Title.
    [DNLM: 1. Joints - physiology - atlases. WE 17 K17p
    1982a]
    QP303.K3613 1982   612'.75   80-42183
    (pbk. :v.2)

 ELSEVIER SCIENCE — your source for books,
journals and multimedia
in the health sciences
www.elsevierhealth.com

Printed in China by RDC Group Limited
B/09

Foreword to the French Edition

This book belongs to a series of three volumes of which the first, on the upper limb, has had well-deserved success.

The same original approach has been adopted in this volume, devoted to the lower limb. The functional anatomy is clearly and precisely set forth with the help of six hundred and ninety diagrams. The explanatory notes on the mechanics of the joints and the physiology of muscle action are at once brief and perfectly clear. This new method makes the study of the anatomy and physiology of joints logical and simple. It will appeal to a wide public ranging from the medical student to the orthopaedic surgeon.

Dr Kapandji should be thanked for devoting his considerable talent as a teacher to the advancement of functional anatomy. There is little doubt that this second volume will be a success.

Doyen Gaston Cordier

Preface to the Fifth Edition

During the last twenty years orthopaedic surgery has been profoundly altered by the advent of prostheses. This second volume is now twenty years old and the fifth editon needed to be modified and improved in the light of modern concepts derived from the prosthesis revolution.

This revised volume has been amended and expanded both in the text and in the illustration section. Fresh material is included in every chapter but particularly in the chapter on the knee, where improvements in clinical examination, arthroscopy and, more recently, the use of scanning devices have led to new ideas about the factors controlling the stability of the joint and hence to new operative procedures. The increasingly complex mechanisms of this joint are not yet fully worked out and the burning question is whether engineers and surgeons will be able to develop ligamentous prostheses, which can be suitably positioned so as to restore joint stability permanently. More detailed knowledge of the bio-mechanics of the knee will undoubtedly provide the answers.

The other chapters have also received due attention. The hip, which appears to be simpler than the knee, can now be better explored with scanning devices. The numerous prostheses in use last only ten to fifteen years and the question arises whether the new uncemented prostheses will last any longer. Here again progress will follow a better understanding of the interaction in space and time of the foreign material and the bone.

Finally, in the chapters devoted to the ankle and the foot are included new data on the instantaneous changes and interaction of the various axes of motion. Stress is laid on the atypical features of these universal joints, which do not conform to their industrial counterparts. The constant flux in the direction and intensity of their mechanical constraints makes it impossible to devise prostheses able to resist the extreme mechanical conditions to which they are subjected.

This fifth edition should thus appeal to old and new readers.

I. A. Kapandji
1987

Contents

The Hip

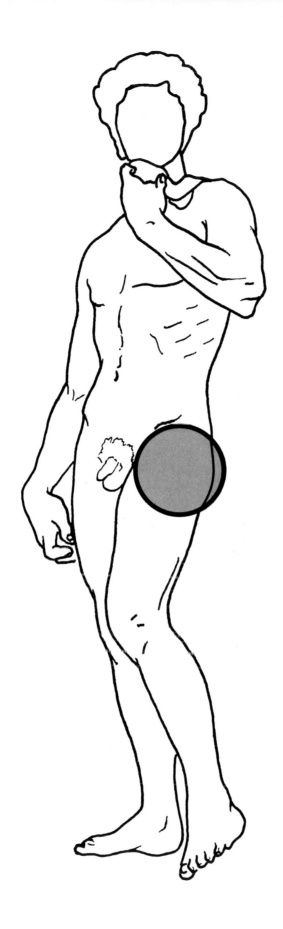

1

MOVEMENTS OF THE HIP AND THEIR RANGES

The hip is the *proximal joint* of the lower limb and, being located at its root, it allows the limb to *assume any position in space*. Hence it has **three axes** and **three degrees of freedom** (fig. 1).

A **transverse** axis XOX', lying in a frontal plane and controlling movements of *flexion and extension*.

An **anteroposterior** axis YOY', lying in a sagittal plane and controlling movements of *adduction and abduction*.

A **vertical** axis OZ, which coincides with the *long axis of the limb* OR when the hip joint is in the 'straight' position. It controls movements of *medial* and *lateral rotation*.

The movements of the hip occur at a single joint: the *hip joint* (coxo-femoral joint). It is a **ball-and-socket joint** with a marked degree of interlocking and in this respect it differs from the shoulder joint which is an open ball-and-socket joint showing great freedom of movement at the expense of stability. The hip joint therefore has a more limited range of movement—partially compensated for by movements of the lumbar vertebral column—but is distinctly *more stable*, being in fact the most difficult joint to dislocate. These features of the hip joint derive from the two basic functions of the lower limb: *support of the body weight* and *locomotion*.

Artificial replacement of the hip ushered in the era of prosthetic surgery, which has revolutionized orthopaedics. With its nearly spherical articular surfaces, the hip is the joint that can be most easily reproduced mechanically, but the protheses are still riddled with problems concerning the proper size of the prosthetic head, the stress coefficient of the surfaces in contact, their resistance to wear, the long-term toxicity of released foreign material and, above all, the mode of contact between prosthesis and acetabulum, whether cemented or not. At present, hip prostheses are the most advanced and the most varied.

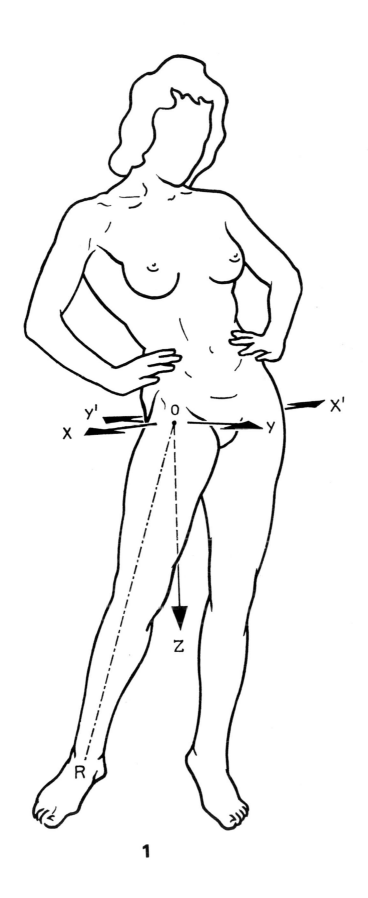

1

MOVEMENTS OF FLEXION OF THE HIP

Flexion of the hip joint is *the movement which approximates the anterior aspect of the thigh to the trunk* so that the whole lower limb comes to lie anterior to the frontal plane, which traverses the joint.

The **range of flexion** varies according to the following conditions:

On the whole, *active* flexion is of lesser range than passive flexion. The *position of the knee joint* also determines the range of flexion: with the knee extended (fig. 2), flexion reaches 90°; with the knee flexed (fig. 3), flexion can reach up to 120° or even beyond.

The range of *passive* flexion always exceeds 120° but is still dependent on the position of the knee. If the knee is extended (fig. 4), the range of flexion is clearly smaller than if the knee is flexed (fig. 5), in the latter case the range exceeds 140° and the thigh is nearly in contact with the thorax. It will be shown later (p. 140) how knee flexion relaxes the hamstrings and allows a greater degree of flexion at the hip.

If both hips undergo passive flexion simultaneously while the knees are flexed (fig. 6), the anterior aspects of the thighs come into contact with the chest. This occurs because flexion of the hip is compounded with posterior tilting of the pelvis due to *flattening of the lumbar curve* (arrowed).

4

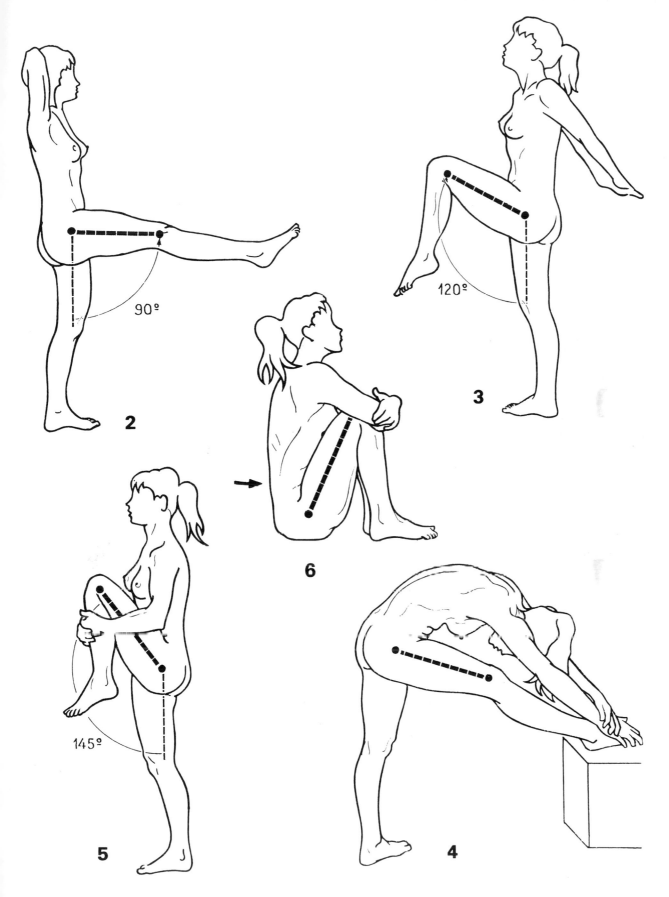

2

90°

3

120°

6

5

145°

4

MOVEMENTS OF EXTENSION OF THE HIP

Extension takes the lower limb posterior to the frontal plane.

The range of extension is notably less than that of flexion and is limited by the tension of the *iliofemoral ligament* (p. 26)

Active extension is of lesser range than passive extension. When the knee is in extension (fig. 7), extension of the hip has a greater range (20°) than when the knee is flexed (fig. 8): this follows from the fact that the hamstrings lose some of their efficiency as extensors of the hip because their contraction has largely been utilised in flexing the knee (p. 140).

Passive extension attains a range of 20° when one bends forwards (fig. 9): it reaches 30° when the lower limb is forcibly pulled back (fig. 10).

Note that extension of the hip is appreciably increased by anterior tilting of the pelvis due to *exaggeration of the lumbar lordosis*. This contribution of the lumbar vertebral column to this movement of extension can be measured (figs. 7 and 8) as the angle between the vertical (fine broken line) and the 'straight' position of the hip (heavy broken line). This 'straight' position is easily determined because the angle between that position of the thigh and the line joining the centre of the hip and the anterosuperior iliac spine is a constant. However, this angle varies with the individual as it *depends upon the orientation of the pelvis*, i.e. the degree of anteroposterior tilting.

The values of the various ranges given apply to the 'normal' untrained subject. They are considerably increased by exercise and training. Ballerinas, for example, commonly do the splits sideways (fig. 11), even, without resting on the ground; this is due to enhanced flexibility of the iliofemoral ligament. However, it is worth noting that they compensate for the inadequate extension of the posterior limb by an appreciable degree of anterior tilting of the pelvis.

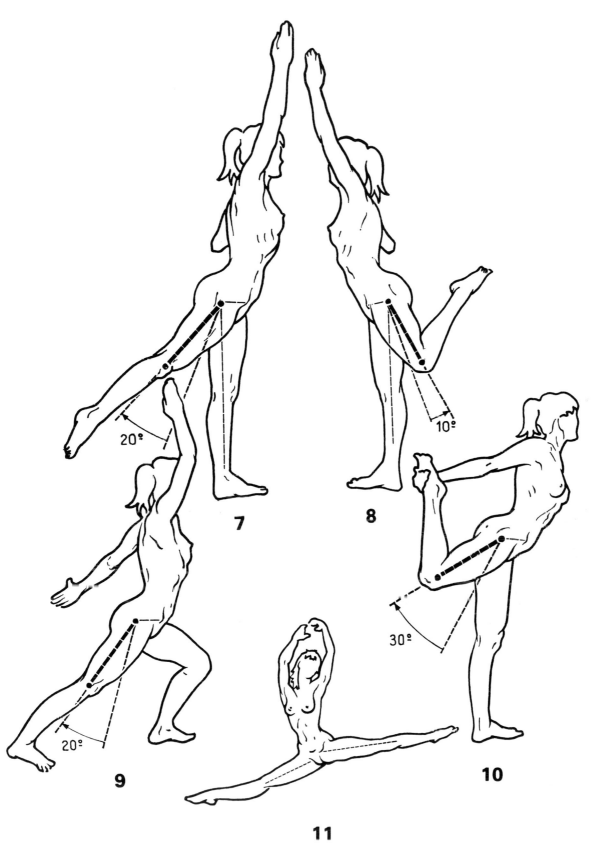

7

8

9

11

10

MOVEMENTS OF ABDUCTION OF THE HIP

Abduction is the movement of the lower limb **directly laterally** and away from the plane of symmetry of the body.

It is theoretically possible to abduct only one hip but *in practice abduction at one joint is automatically followed by a similar degree of abduction at the other joint*. This becomes obvious after 30° abduction (fig. 12), when one first clearly notices tilting of the pelvis, as judged from the displacement of the line joining the surface markings of the two posterior iliac spines. If the long axes of the lower limbs are produced they intersect on the line of symmetry of the pelvis. This indicates that in this position each limb has been abducted 15°.

When **abduction reaches a maximum** (fig. 13), the angle between the two lower limbs is a right angle. Once more abduction can be seen to have occurred symmetrically at both joints so that each limb has a maximum of 45° abduction. The pelvis is now tilted at an angle of 45° to the horizontal and 'looks' towards the supporting limb. The vertebral column as a whole makes up for this pelvic tilt by bending laterally towards the supporting side. Here too the vertebral column is seen to *be involved in movements of the hip*.

Abduction is checked by the impact of the femoral neck on the acetabular rim (p. 22), but before this occurs it has usually been restrained by the adductor muscles and the ilio- and pubofemoral ligaments (p. 30).

Training can notably augment the maximal range of abduction, e.g. ballerinas who can achieve 120° (fig. 14) to 130° (fig. 15) of *active* abduction without any support. For *passive* abduction trained subjects can attain 180° abduction *by doing the splits sideways* (fig. 16, a). In fact, this is no longer pure abduction since, to slacken the iliofemoral ligaments, the pelvis is tilted anteriorly (fig. 16, b) while the lumbar vertebral column is hyperextended i.e. the hip is now in a position of abduction and flexion.

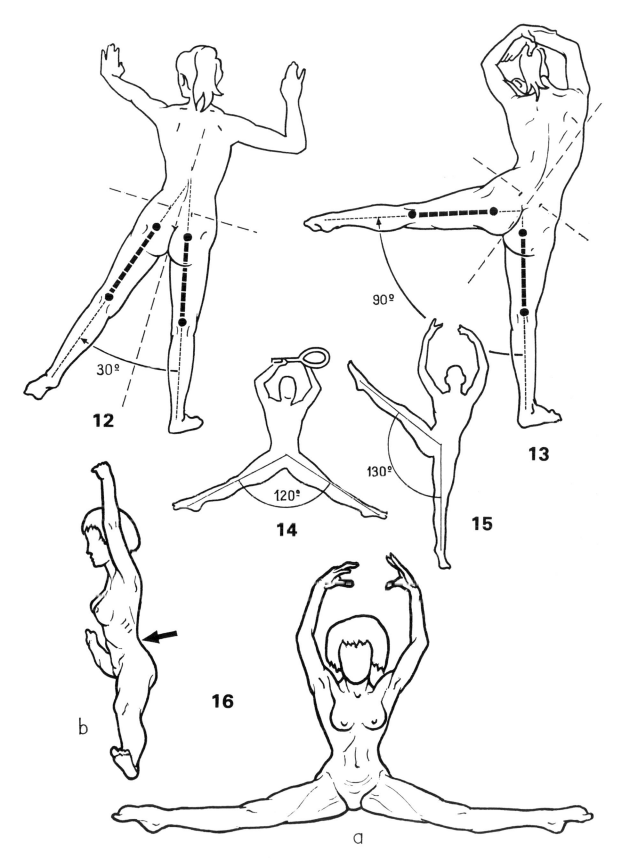

12

90°

30°

13

120°

14

130°

15

16

b

a

9

MOVEMENTS OF ADDUCTION OF THE HIP

Adduction is the movement of the lower limb **medially** towards the plane of symmetry of the body. As in the position of reference both limbs are in contact, there is no *pure adduction*.

On the other hand, **relative adduction** exists as when the limb moves medially from any position of abduction (fig. 17).

There are also movements of **combined adduction and extension** (fig. 18) and of **combined adduction and flexion** at the hip (fig. 19). Finally there are **movements of adduction at one hip combined with abduction at the other hip** (fig. 20); these are associated with tilting of the pelvis and bending of the vertebral column. Note that when the feet are set apart—this is necessary to maintain one's balance—the angle of adduction at one hip is not equal to that of abduction at the other (fig. 21). The difference between these two angles is equal to the angle between the two axes of the lower limbs as they lie in the initial position of symmetry.

In all these combined movements involving adduction the *maximal range of adduction is 30°*.

Of all these combined movements, one happens to be very common, as illustrated by the position of a person sitting with legs crossed (fig. 22). Adduction is then associated with flexion and external rotation. This is the position of *maximal instability* for the hip (p. 36).

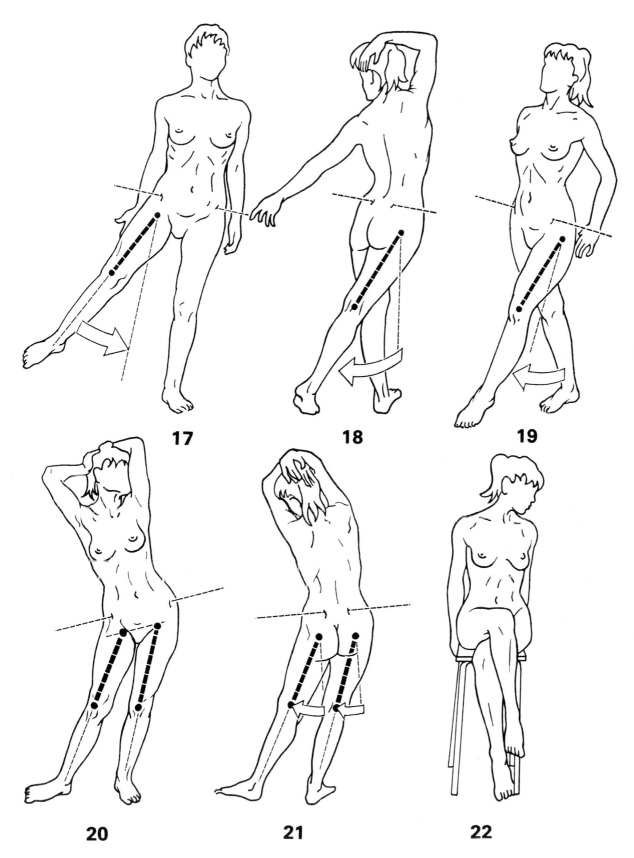

17

18

19

20

21

22

ROTATIONAL MOVEMENTS OF THE HIP

These occur about the *mechanical axis* of the lower limb (axis OR, fig. 1). In the 'straight' position this axis coincides with the vertical axis of the hip (axis OZ, fig. 1). Under these circumstances, **lateral rotation** is the movement of the limb that brings the tips of the toes to face outwards and **medial rotation** brings the tips of the toes to face inwards. As the knee is fully extended, rotation occurs only at the hip (p. 126).

However, this is not the position used for assessing the range of rotational movements. This is more easily done with the subject lying prone or sitting on the edge of a table with his knee flexed at 90°.

When the subject is *lying prone*, the **position of reference** (fig. 23) is achieved when the leg is at right angles to the thigh and is *vertical*. From this position, when the leg moves *laterally*, **medial rotation** occurs with a total range of 30° to 40° (fig. 24); when the leg moves *medially*, **lateral rotation** (fig. 25) occurs with a total range of 60°.

When the subject is *sitting on the edge of a table* with the hip and knee flexed at 90° the same criteria apply: when the leg moves medially, *lateral rotation* (fig. 26) takes place and when the leg moves laterally *medial rotation* (fig. 27) takes place. In this position the total range of lateral rotation can be *greater* than in the lying position because hip flexion relaxes the ilio- and pubofemoral ligaments, which play a vital part in checking lateral rotation (p. 30).

In the squatting position (fig. 28) lateral rotation is combined with abduction and flexion exceeding 90°. Yoga experts can achieve such a degree of lateral rotation that the two legs become parallel and horizontal ('position of the lotus').

The range of rotation depends on the angle of anteversion of the femoral neck, which is usually quite wide in the child. This leads to *medial rotation of the thigh* and the walking child displays a bilateral genu valgum and a talipes planivalgus. With growth this angle of anteversion decreases to normal adult values and these walking problems begin to disappear. This wide angle of anteversion, however, can be maintained and even increased when children become accustomed to *sitting on the ground with their heels pressed against each other* and their hips flexed. This posture causes medial rotation of the femur and accentuates the angle of anteversion as a result of the great plasticity of the young skeleton. This defect can be corrected by forcing the child to adopt the inverse sitting position, i.e. *the squatting position* or, even better, the *'lotus position.'* With time this leads to remodelling of the femoral neck in a more retroverted position.

This angle of anteversion was difficult to measure by routine radiology but with computed tomography it can be measured easily and accurately. The scanner should thus be used to evaluate malrotations of the lower limb, which usually 'start' at the hip.

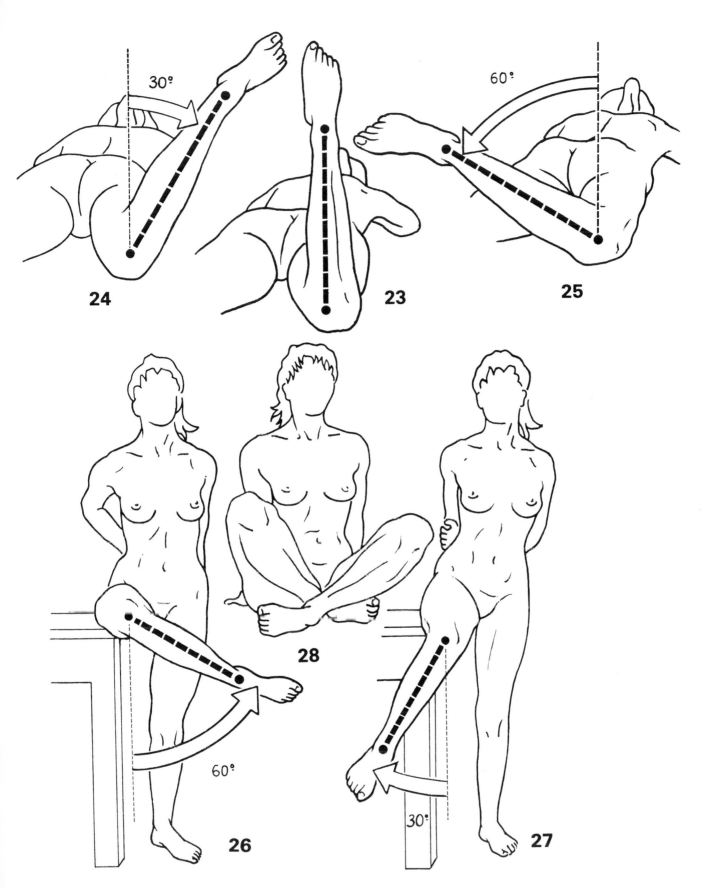

24

23

25

28

26

60°

27

30°

13

MOVEMENTS OF CIRCUMDUCTION OF THE HIP

As with all joints possessing three degrees of freedom, the movement of circumduction of the hip is defined as **the combination of the elementary movements occurring simultaneously around the three axes.** When circumduction is of maximal range, the axis of the lower limb traces in space a cone with its apex lying at the centre of the hip: this is the **cone of circumduction** (fig. 29).

This cone is far from symmetrical as the maximal ranges of the various elementary movements in space are not equal. The path traced by the extremity of the lower limb is not a circle but an irregular curve traversing the various sectors of space established by the intersection of the three planes of reference:

    A. Sagittal plane containing movments of flexion and extension;

    B. Frontal plane containing movements of abduction and adduction;

    C. Horizontal plane.

The eight sectors of space are numbered I to VIII and the cone traverses successively the following sectors: III, II, I, IV, V and VIII. (Sector VIII lies below plane C, diagonally opposite sector IV.) Note how the curve skirts the supporting limb; if the latter were removed the curve would reach further medially. The arrow R which represents the distal, anterior and lateral prolongation of the lower limb in sector IV is the **axis of the cone of circumduction** and corresponds to *the position of function and of immobilisation of the hip.*

Strasser has suggested that this curve should be inscribed on a sphere (fig. 30) with centre O lying at the centre of the hip joint, with radius OL equal to the length of the femur and with Eq representing the equator. On this sphere, one can determine the various range maxima with the use of a system of latitudes and longitudes (not shown in the diagram).

He has proposed also a similar method for the shoulder joint, where it is more applicable because of the greater degree of longitudinal rotation of the upper limb.

Starting from an arbitrary position OL of the femur, movements of abduction (arrow Ab) and of abduction (arrow Ad) occur along the horizontal meridian (HM); movements of medial rotation (arrow MR) and lateral rotation (arrow LR) take place about the axis OL. Movements of flexion and extension fall into two groups depending on whether they occur along a parallel P (flexion F_1, then called circumpolar) or along the large circle C (flexion F_2, then called circumcentral). These distinctions are of little practical value.

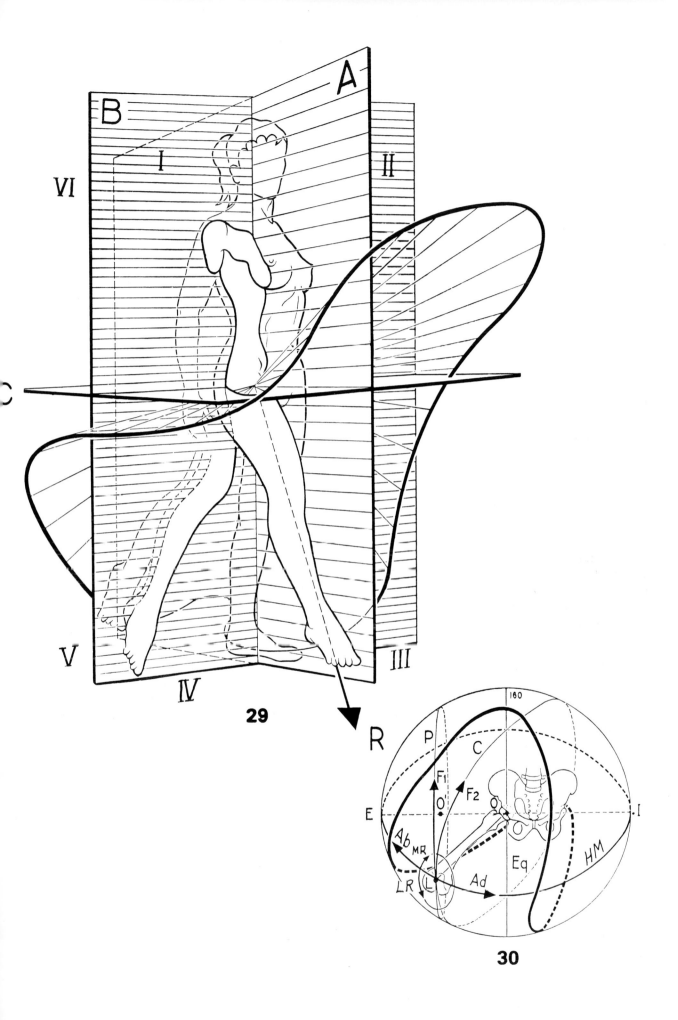

29

30

ORIENTATION OF THE FEMORAL HEAD AND ACETABULUM
(the numbers are common to all the diagrams)

The hip is of the **ball-and-socket variety** with **spherical** articular surfaces.

The **femoral head** (fig. 31, seen from in front) forms about two-thirds of a sphere of diameter 4 to 5 cm. Its geometrical centre is traversed by the three axes of the joint: horizontal axis (1), vertical axis (2), antero-posterior axis (3). The head is supported by the neck of the femur which joins the shaft. The axis of the femoral neck is obliquely set and runs superiorly, medially and anteriorly. In the adult it forms an obtuse angle of 125° with the femoral shaft (D) and an acute angle of 10° to 30° with the frontal plane (fig. 37, seen from above); this angle faces medially and anteriorly and is also called the *angle of anteversion*. Therefore (fig. 34, seen from behind and from inside) the coronal plane through the centre of the femoral head and the axis of the femoral condyles (plane P) lies almost completely *anterior* to the femoral shaft and its upper extremity. *This plane P contains the mechanical axis MM' of the lower limb and this axis forms an angle of 5° to 7° with the axis of the shaft (D)* (p. 66).

The shape of the head and neck varies considerably with the individual and, according to anthropologists, it is the result of functional adaptation. Two extreme types are described (fig. 35, according to Bellugue):—

Type I: the head is more than two-thirds of a sphere, the angle between the neck and the shaft (I = 125°) and that between the neck and the frontal plane (D = 25°) are maximal. The shaft is slender and the pelvis is small and high slung. Such a configuration favours range of movement at the joint and corresponds to an adaptation to speed of movement (fig. 35, a and c).

Type II: the head just exceeds a hemisphere, the angles (I = 115°, D = 10°) are minimal. The shaft is thicker and the pelvis large and broad. The range of movement is reduced and the loss of speed is made up for by the greater strength of the joint. This is the configuration 'of power'.

The **acetabulum** (fig. 32; seen from lateral aspect) receives the femoral head and lies on the lateral aspect of the hip bone where its three constituent bones meet. It is hemispherical and is bounded by the acetabular rim (R). Only the sides of the acetabulum are lined by a *horseshoe-shaped articular cartilage* (Ca), which is interrupted inferiorly by the deep *acetabular notch*. The central part of the cavity is deeper than the articular cartilage and is non-articular: it is called the *acetabular fossa* (Af) and is separated from the inner face of the pelvic bone by a thin plate of bone (fig. 33; transparent bone). It will be shown later (p. 22) how the *labrum acetabulare* is applied to the acetabular rim.

The acetabulum is directed *laterally, inferiorly and anteriorly* (arrow C' representing the axis of the acetabulum). A vertical section of the acetabulum (fig. 36) shows quite clearly that it faces inferiorly: the acetabular axis forms an angle of 30° to 40° with the horizontal, so that the upper part of the acetabulum 'overhangs' the femoral head laterally. This degree of overhanging is measured by the angle W (Wiberg), which is normally 30°. The roof of the cavity sustains the greatest pressure from the femoral head and so the articular cartilage of the acetabulum and of the femoral head is thickest superiorly.

The horizontal section (fig. 37) shows the anterior orientation of the acetabulum: the axis C' is at an angle of 30° to 40° with the frontal plane. Also included are: the acetabular fossa (Af) lying deep to the articular cartilage (Ca); the labrum acetabulare (LA) continuous with the acetabular rim (AR); the plane tangential to the rim, which runs obliquely anteriorly and medially.

In practice these sections of the joint can be obtained as follows:

for the vertical section, **tomography** gives a picture close to figure 36.

for the horizontal section, **computed tomography** of the hip gives a picture close to figure 37 and allows the angle of anteversion of the acetabulum and of the femoral neck to be measured. These measurements can be useful in the diagnosis of hip dysplasias.

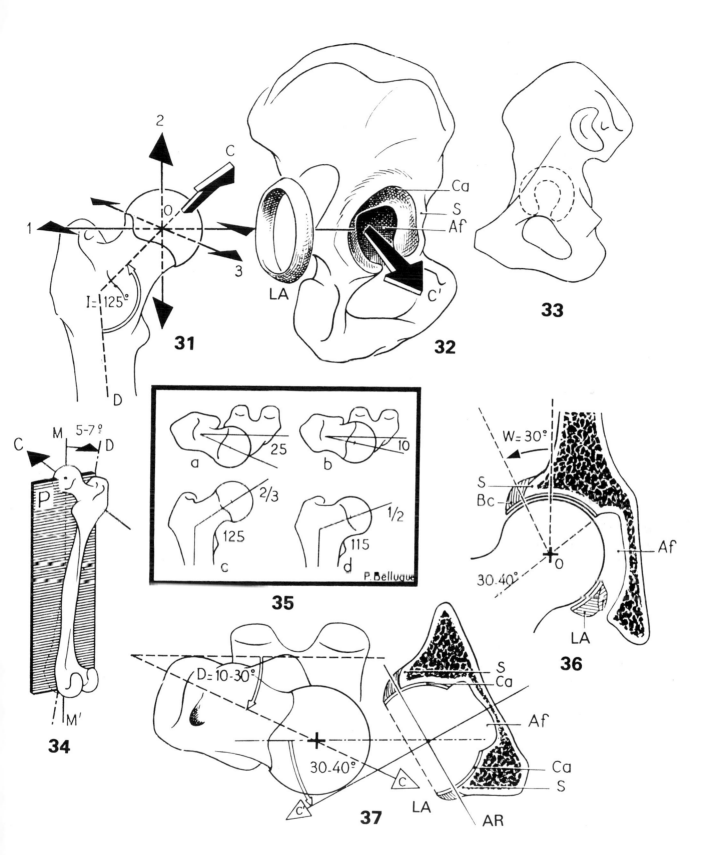

RELATIONSHIPS OF THE ARTICULAR SURFACES

When the hip is in **the 'neutral' position** (fig. 38), which corresponds to *the erect posture* (fig. 39), the femoral head is not completely covered by the acetabulum, the cartilage-lined anterosuperior aspect being exposed (arrowed fig. 38). This results (fig. 44, three-dimensional diagram of the axes of the right hip) from the fact that the axis of the femoral neck (C), which runs obliquely superiorly, anteriorly and medially, is out of line with the acetabular axis (C′), which runs obliquely inferiorly, *anteriorly* and laterally. A mechanical model of the hip (fig. 40) illustrates this arrangement as follows: a sphere is fixed to a shaft so as to mimic the femoral head and neck; the plane D represents the plane passing through the axis of the femoral shaft, and the transverse axis of the femoral condyles. On the other hand, a hemisphere is suitably arranged in relation to the sagittal plane S; the plane F represents the frontal plane passing through the centre of the hemisphere. In the 'straight' position, the sphere is largely exposed superiorly and anteriorly: the black crescent represents the portion of articular cartilage which is exposed.

By moving the 'acetabular hemisphere' and the 'femoral sphere' (fig. 43) one can achieve complete coincidence of the articular surfaces with disappearance of the exposed 'black crescent'. Thanks to the planes of reference S and P, it is clear that this coincidence is brought about by *three elementary movements*:

flexion of approximately 90° (arrow 1);

a small measure of abduction (arrow 2);

a small measure of lateral rotation (arrow 3).

In this position the axis of the acetabulum (C′) and that of the femoral neck (C″) are in line (fig. 45).

On the skeleton (fig. 41), coincidence of the articular surfaces is achieved by the same movements of flexion, abduction and lateral rotation so that the head lies completely within the acetabular cavity. This position of the hip corresponds to the *position on all fours* (fig. 42), which is therefore the *true physiological position of the hip*. During evolution, the transition from the quadruped to the biped state has led to **the loss of coincidence of the articular surfaces of the hip joint.** Conversely, this lack of coincidence of these articular surfaces can be considered as an argument in favour of man's origin from quadruped ancestors.

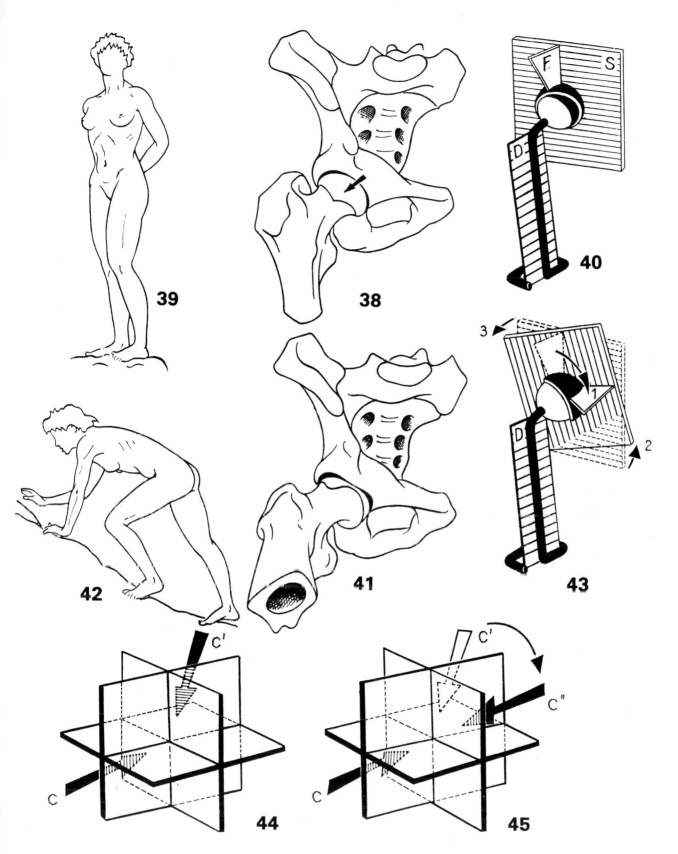

39

38

40

42

41

43

44

45

THE STRUCTURE OF THE FEMUR AND PELVIS

The head, neck and shaft of the femur can be compared to the structure known as an *'overhang'* in engineering. In fact, the weight of the body, when applied to the femoral head, is transmitted to the shaft *by a lever arm*, the femoral neck. A similar set-up is seen in the *gibbet* (fig. 50), where the weight acting vertically tends to 'shear' the horizontal beam near its junction with the shaft and so to close the angle between the two. To prevent this occurrence a *strut* is interposed obliquely.

The femoral head represents the horizontal beam of the gibbet and an overall picture (fig. 48) of the lower limb shows that the mechanical axis of its three joints (heavy broken line) runs medial to the femoral head (n.b. the mechanical axis does not coincide with the vertical shown by the line of alternate dashes and dots). The mechanical significance of this arrangement will emerge later (fig. 128).

To prevent the shearing of the base of the femoral head (fig. 51) the **upper end of the femur** has a special structural pattern which can be easily seen in a *vertical section* of the desiccated bone (fig. 46). The lamellae of spongy bone are arranged in *two systems of trabeculae* corresponding to the *lines of force*.

The **main system** consists of two sets of trabeculae fanning out into neck and head:

1. the *first set* (1) arises from the cortical layer of the lateral aspect of the femoral shaft and terminates on the inferior aspect of the cortical layer of the femoral head (the so-called *arcuate bundle* of Gallois and Bosquette).

2. the *second set* (2), arising from the cortex of the internal aspect of the shaft and of the inferior part of the neck, fans out vertically in an upward direction to terminate on the cortical bone of the superior aspect of the head (the so-called *'supporting bundle'*).

Culmann has shown experimentally that, when a test bar is loaded and bent into the shape of a crook or a crane (fig. 49), this gives rise to two sets of lines of force: an oblique set, appearing on the convex aspect, which corresponds to the *shearing stresses* and is the counterpart of the arcuate bundle; a vertical set, lying in the concavity which corresponds to *compressive forces* and is the counterpart of the 'supporting bundle' (the strut of the gibbet).

The **accessory system**, consists of two bundles which fan out into the greater trochanter:

the *first bundle* (3), arising from the cortical layer of the inner aspect of the shaft (*trochanteric bundle*);

the *second bundle* (4) (less important), consisting of vertical trabeculae running parallel to the greater trochanter.

Three points are worth noting:

1. In the greater trochanter the arcuate bundle (1) and the trochanteric bundle (3) intersect to form a *Gothic arch* and its *keystone*, running down from the superior aspect of the neck, consists of much denser bone. The inner pillar (3) is less strong and weakens with age as a result of senile osteoporosis.

2. The neck and head also contain *another Gothic arch* formed by the intersection of the arcuate bundle (1) and the supporting bundle (2). At the point of intersection the bone is denser and constitutes the *'nucleus of the head'*. This system of trabeculae rests on an extremely strong support, the thick cortical layer of the inferior aspect of the neck, known as the inferior spur of the neck (SP) or else as the vault of Adams.

3. Between the Gothic arch of the trochanter and the supporting bundle is a *zone of weakness* (+), which is intensified by senile osteoporosis: it is the site of basal fractures of the neck (fig. 51).

The *structure of the pelvis* (fig. 46) can also be studied in the same way. Since it constitutes a closed ring, it transmits vertical forces from the vertebral column (horizontally striped double arrow) to the two hip joints.

There are two main *trabecular systems* that transmit the stresses from the sacro-iliac joint to the *acetabulum* on the one hand and the *ischium* on the other (figs. 46 and 47).

The **sacro-acetabular trabeculae** fall into two sets:

1. The first set (5), arising from the upper part of the acetabulum, converges ont eh posterior border of the greater sciatic notch to form the 'sciatic spur' (SS). It is thence reflected laterally before fanning out towards the inferior aspect of the acetabulum, where it falls into line with the lines of force (traction) of the femoral neck (1).

2. The second set (6) arises from the inferior part of the acetabulum and converges on to the level of the superior gluteal line to form the 'innominate spine' (IS). From there it is reflected laterally and fans out towards the upper aspect of the acetabulum, where it falls into line with the lines of force (compression) of the femoral neck (2).

The **sacro-ischial trabeculae** (7) arise from the acetabulum in conjunction with the above-mentioned bundles and then run downwards to the ischium. They intersect the trabeculae arising from the acetabular rim (8). These trabeculae bear the body weight in the sitting position.

Finally, the trabeculae arising from the innominate spine (IS) and the 'sciatic spur' run together into the horizontal ramus of the pubis to complete the pelvic ring.

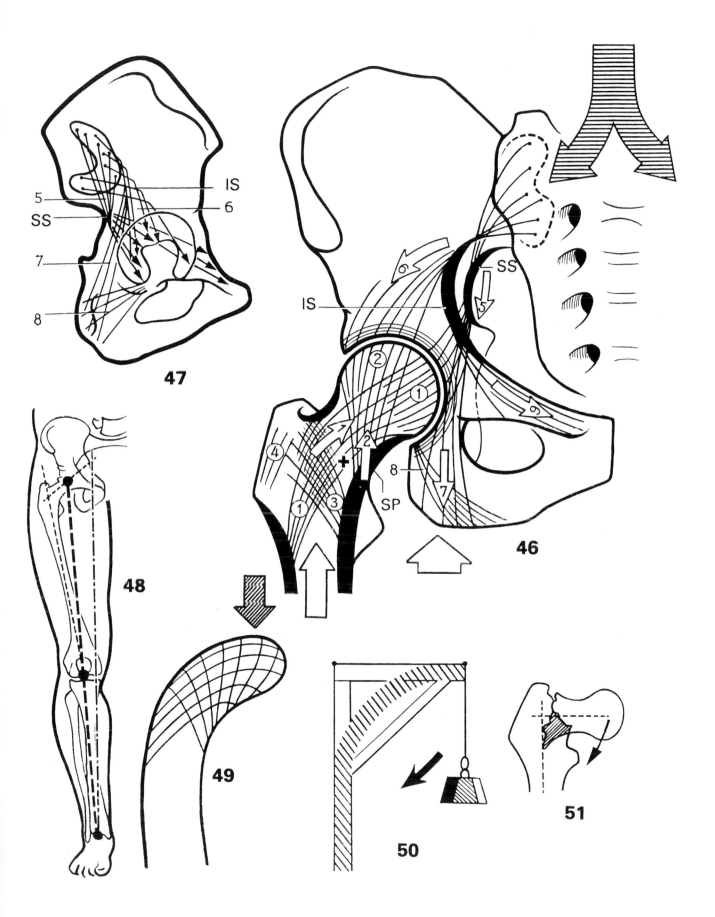

47

IS
5
SS
6
7
8

46

SS
IS
6
2
1
5
4
+
2
1
3
8
SP
7
9

48

49

50

51

THE LABRUM ACETABULARE AND THE LIGAMENTUM TERES OF THE FEMORAL HEAD

The **labrum acetabulare** (LA) is a **fibrocartilaginous ring** inserted into the acetabular rim (fig. 52). It deepens the acetabulum considerably (p. 36) and fills out the various gaps of the acetabular rim (R). The anterosuperior aspect of the labrum has been removed and shows the 'iliopubic notch' (IPN). The ischiopubic or *acetabular notch* (AN), which is the deepest of the three notches, is bridged by the labrum as it gains insertion into the *transverse acetabular ligament* (TAL) which is itself inserted into the two sides of the notch. (The diagram shows the ligament and labrum 'displaced'.) The section (fig. 53) shows the labrum well fixed to the edge of the notch and to the transverse ligament (see also fig. 36).

The labrum is in fact **triangular** on section and possesses **three surfaces**: an *internal* surface which is completely inserted into the acetabular rim and the transverse ligament; a *central* surface (looking into the joint), which is lined by articular cartilage continuous with that of the acetabulum and consequently articulates with the femoral head; a *peripheral* surface which receives the attachment of the joint capsule (C) only at its base so that the sharp edge of the labrum lies free within the joint cavity and a circular recess (CR) is formed between the labrum and the capsular attachment (fig. 54, according to Rouvière).

The **ligamentum teres** (LT) of the femoral head (fig. 56) is a flattened fibrous band 3 to 3·5 cm. long, which arises from the acetabular notch (fig. 52) and runs on the floor of the acetabular fossa (fig. 53) before its insertion into the *fovea femoris capitis* (fig. 55). This fovea lies slightly inferior and posterior to the centre of the articular surface of the head. The ligament is inserted into the anterosuperior part of the fovea and only glides in contact with its inferior surface. The ligament consists of *three bundles* (fig. 56):

the *posterior ischial bundle* (pi) (the longest), which runs through the acetabular notch under the transverse ligament (fig. 52) to be inserted below and behind the posterior horn of the horseshoe articular crescent;

the *anterior pubic bundle* (ap), which is inserted into the acetabular notch itself behind the anterior horn of the articular crescent;

the *intermediate bundle* (ib) (the thinnest), which is inserted into the upper border of the transverse ligament (fig. 52).

The ligamentum teres (fig. 53) lies embedded in fibro-adipose tissue within the acetabular fossa (AF) and is lined by synovium (fig. 54). The synovial lining is attached on the one hand to the central aspect of the articular crescent and the upper aspect of the transverse ligament, and on the other to the femoral head around the fovea. It therefore has roughly the shape of a truncated cone, hence its name of 'tent of the ligamentum teres' (Ts).

The ligamentum teres plays only a trivial mechanical role though it is extremely strong (breaking force equivalent to 45 kg. weight). However, it contributes to the *vascular supply of the femoral head*. The posterior branch of the obturator artery (1) (fig. 57: seen from below, according to Rouvière) sends off a tiny branch—*the artery of the ligamentum teres* (6)—which runs underneath the transverse ligament before entering the ligament. The head and neck also receive an arterial supply from the capsular vessels (5) arising from the medial (3) and lateral (4) circumflex arteries (branches of the profunda (2)).

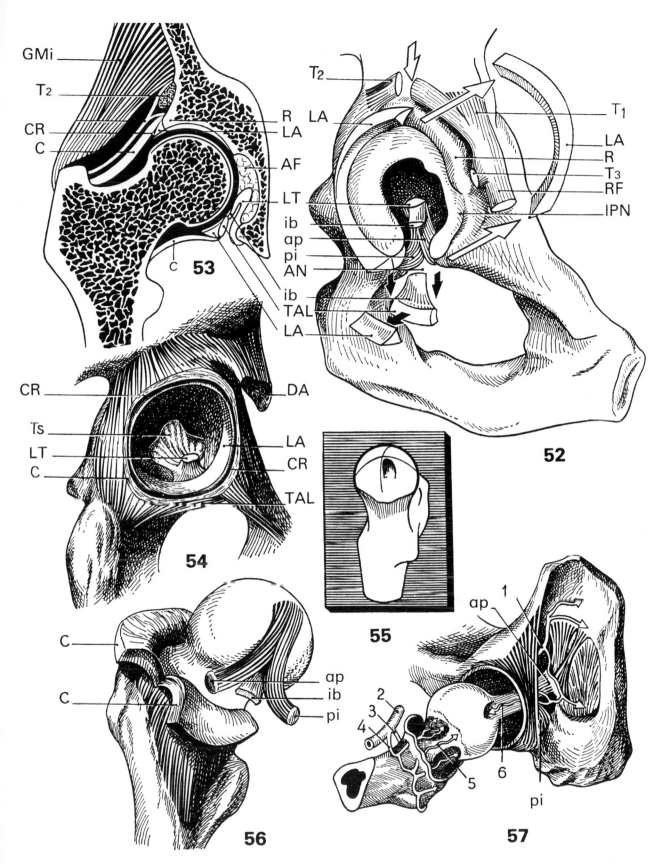

GMi

T₂

CR

C

R
LA
AF
LT
ib
ap
pi
AN
ib
TAL
LA

c **53**

T₂
LA

52

T₁
LA
R
T₃
RF
IPN

CR

Ts
LT
C

DA

LA
CR
TAL

54

55

C

C

ap
ib
pi

56

1
ap

2
3
4
5
6
pi

57

23

THE CAPSULAR LIGAMENT OF THE HIP

The capsule is shaped like a **cylindrical sleeve**, (fig. 58) running from the iliac bone to the upper end of the femur. It is made up of *four distinct sets of fibres*:

longitudinal fibres (1), which help to unite the articular surfaces and run parallel to the axis of the cylinder;

oblique fibres (2), of similar function to that of (1), form a spiral round the cylinder;

arcuate fibres (3), attached only to the hip bone. They run in a criss-cross fashion from one end of the acetabular rim to the other and form an arc of varying height and apex flush with the middle of the sleeve. These arcuate fibres are arranged like a man's tie around the femoral head and help to keep it within the acetabulum;

circular fibres (4) with no bony attachments. They are particularly abundant in the middle of the sleeve which they groove slightly. They stand out on the deep surface of the capsule and are known as the *zona orbicularis* (the ring of Weber), which surrounds the neck.

Medially, the capsular ligament is inserted into the acetabular rim (5), the transverse ligament and the peripheral surface of the labrum (p. 22). It is intimately related to the tendon of the rectus femoris (RF, fig. 52) as follows:—

The *straight head* (T_1) of the rectus femoris arising from the antero-inferior iliac spine, and the *reflected head* (T_2), arising from the groove above the rim of the acetabulum, unite before running between the two slips of the capsular insertion (fig. 53) reinforced superiorly by the ilio-femoral ligament (p. 26). The *deep recurrent fibres* (T_3) strengthen the anterior aspect of the capsule.

Laterally, the capsule is not inserted into the edges of the articular cartilage but at the base of the neck along a line which runs:

anteriorly (fig. 58), along *the trochanteric line* (6);

posteriorly (fig. 59), not along trochanteric crest (7), but at the junction of the lateral and middle thirds of the femoral neck (8), just above the *groove* (9) of the obturator externus before its insertion into the trochanteric fossa (TF).

The line of insertion of the capsule is oblique to both the inferior and superior surfaces of the neck. Inferiorly (10), it runs superior and about 1·5 cm. anterior to the lesser trochanter (Lt). The deepest fibres extend up the lower surface of the neck to reach the edge of the cartilage and in so doing they raise synovial folds (*frenula capsulae* (11)), the longest of which is the *pectinofoveal fold of Amantini* (12).

These frenula capsulae are useful during movements of abduction. During adduction (fig. 60) the inferior part of the capsule (1) slackens while the upper part becomes taut (2). During abduction (fig. 61) the frenula (3) unpleat and, by increasing the length of the inferior part of the capsule, enhance the range of the movement: the upper part of the capsule is thrown into folds (2) while the neck impacts on to the acetabular rim via the labrum which becomes distorted and everted (4). This explains why the *labrum deepens the acetabulum without limiting movements at the joint*.

In extreme flexion the anterosuperior aspect of the neck comes into contact with the acetabular rim and in some individuals (fig. 58) the neck at this point bears an iliac impression (II) just above the edge of the articular cartilage.

After injection of a radio-opaque medium into the hip, **arthographic pictures** can be obtained showing the following features (fig. 62):

the *zona orbicularis* (9) indents the capsule distinctly in the middle and divides the joint cavity into two chambers: a *lateral* (1) and a *medial* (2) chamber. These two chambers form the *superior recesses* (3) above and the *inferior recesses* (4) below. The medial chamber also contains:

above, a spur-like recess with its apex pointing towards the acetabular rim, the so-called *supralimbic recess* (5) (compare with fig. 53);

below, two rounded peninsulae separated by a deep gulf: these are respectively the *two acetabular recesses* (6) and the capsular impression of the *ligamentum teres* (7).

Finally can be seen the *interspace* (8) between the femoral head and the acetabulum.

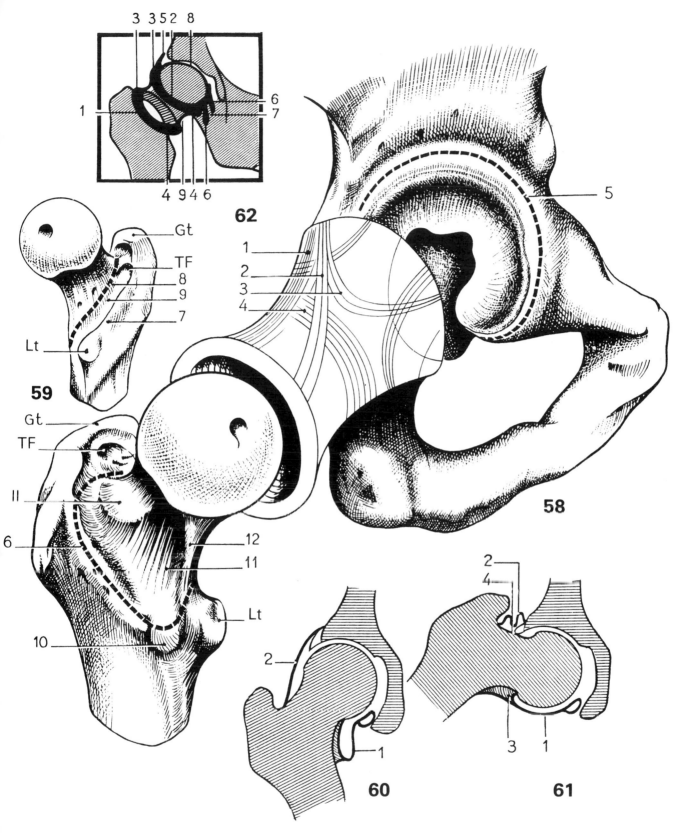

3 3 5 2 8

1

6
7

4 9 4 6

62

5

1
2
3
4

58

Gt
TF
8
9
7
Lt

59

Gt
TF
II
6
10

12
11
Lt

2

2
4

3 1

60

61

THE LIGAMENTS OF THE HIP
(the numbers refer to the same structures in all the diagrams)

The capsule of the hip is strengthened by powerful ligaments anteriorly and posteriorly.

Anteriorly two ligaments are present (fig. 63):

the **iliofemoral ligament** (ligament of Bertin) (1), fan-shaped with its apex attached to the lower part of the antero-inferior iliac spine (site of origin of the rectus femoris, RF) and its base inserted into the whole length of the trochanteric line. Its central part (c) is relatively thin and weak while its two borders are strengthened by:

the *iliotrochanteric or superior band* (a) which is the strongest of the ligaments of the joint, being 8 to 10 mm. thick. It is attached laterally to the upper part of the trochanteric line. It is itself strengthened superiorly by another ligament, called the *ilio-tendino-trochanteric ligament* (d), which according to Rouvière is formed by the fusion of the deep recurrent fibres of the rectus femoris (e) and of a fibrous band arising from the acetabular rim (f). The deep surface of the gluteus minimus (GMi) sends off an aponeurotic expansion (g) which blends with the external aspect of the iliotrochanteric ligament;

the *inferior band* (b) which has the same site of origin as the former and is inserted laterally into the lower part of the trochanteric line.

The **pubofemoral ligament** (2) is attached medially to the anterior aspect of the iliopubic eminence, the superior ramus of the pubic bone and the obturator crest where its fibres blend with those of the pectineus muscle. It is inserted laterally into the anterior surface of the trochanteric fossa.

Taken as a whole (fig. 64), these two ligaments, lying in front of the hip joint, resemble the letter N (Welcker) or better the letter Z with its superior limb (a), i.e. the iliotrochanteric band, lying almost horizontally, its middle limb (b), i.e. the inferior band, running nearly vertically and its inferior limb (2), i.e. the pubofermoral ligament, lying horizontal. Between the pubofemoral ligament and the iliofemoral ligament (+), the capsule is thinner and is related to the bursa intervening between the capsule and the iliopsoas tendon (IP). Occasionally the capsule is perforated at the level and the joint cavity communicates with the iliopsoas bursa.

Posteriorly (fig. 65) there is only one ligament:

the **ischiofermoral ligament** (3) arises from the posterior surface of the acetabular rim and the labrum. Its fibres, running superiorly and laterally, cross the posterior aspect of the neck (h) and gain insertion into the inner surface of the greater trochanter anterior to the trochanteric fossa, where is also inserted the tendon of the obturator externus after traversing the groove lining the capsular insertion (white arrow). Figure 66 also shows some of its fibres (i) which blend directly with the zona orbicularis (j).

As man evolved from the quadruped posture to the erect posture and the pelvis became tilted posteriorly (p. 18), all the ligaments became *coiled* round the femoral neck in the same direction. Figure 67 (right hip, seen from the outside) shows that the ligaments run in a clockwise direction from the hip bone to the femur, i.e. *extension winds these ligaments* round the neck and *flexion unwinds them.*

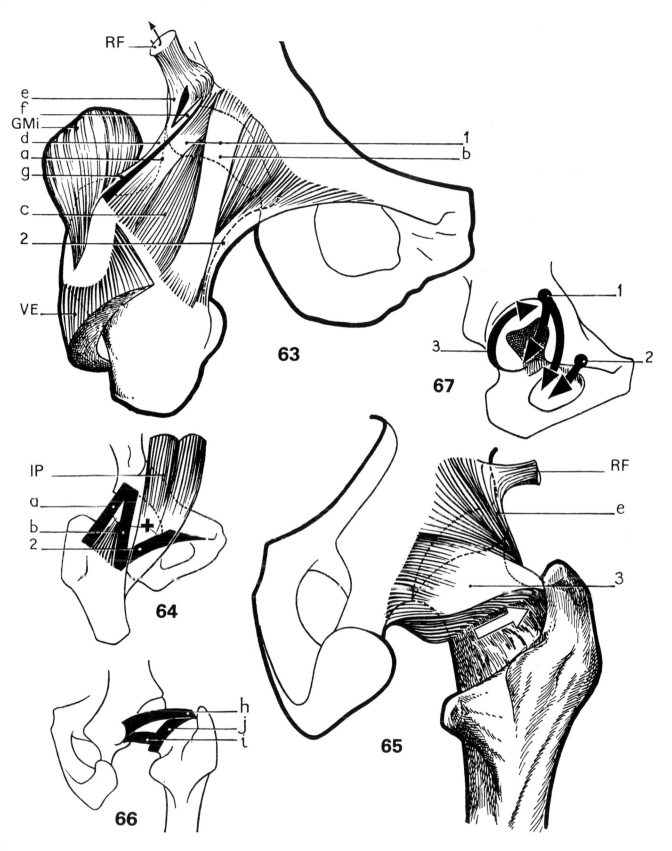

63

RF
e
f
GMi
d
a
g
c
2
VE

67
1
3
2

64
IP
a
b
2

65
RF
e
3

66
h
j
i

27

ROLE OF THE LIGAMENTS IN FLEXION AND EXTENSION

In **the erect position** (fig. 68) the ligaments are under *moderate tension*. This is diagrammatically illustrated in figure 69, where the ring represents the acetabulum and the circle in the centre the femoral head and neck, the ligaments, drawn in as springs, run between the ring and the circle. The iliofemoral ligament (ILF) and the ischiofemoral ligament (ISF) are also included (for simplicity's sake the pubofemoral ligament is not included).

During **extension of the hip** (fig. 70) all the *ligaments become taut* as they wind round the femoral neck (fig. 71). Of all these ligaments the *inferior band of the iliofemoral ligament* is under the greatest tension as it runs nearly vertically (fig. 70) and so is responsible for checking the posterior tilt of the pelvis.

During **flexion of the hip** (fig. 72) the opposite holds good and *all the ligaments without exception are relaxed* (fig. 73).

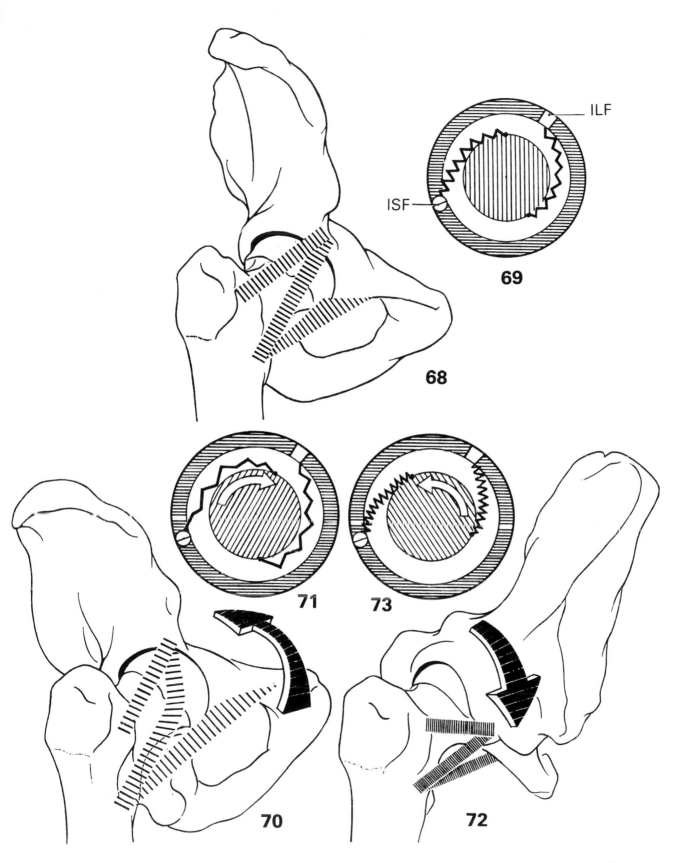

ILF

ISF

69

68

71   **73**

70   **72**

29

ROLE OF THE LIGAMENTS IN LATERAL AND MEDIAL ROTATION

During **lateral rotation of the hip** (fig. 74) the trochanteric line moves away from the acetabular rim with the result that *all the anterior ligaments of the hip become taut* and especially those bands running horizontally, i.e. the **iliotrochanteric band and pubofemoral ligament**. This tightening of the anterior ligaments is well demonstrated in a horizontal section seen from above (fig. 75) and in a postero-superior view of the joint (fig. 76). These also show that during lateral rotation the *ischio-femoral ligament is slackened*.

During **medial rotation** (fig. 77) the converse obtains: *all the anterior ligaments become slack,* especially the iliotrochanteric band and the pubofemoral ligament whereas the *ischiofemoral ligament tenses up* (figs. 78 and 79).

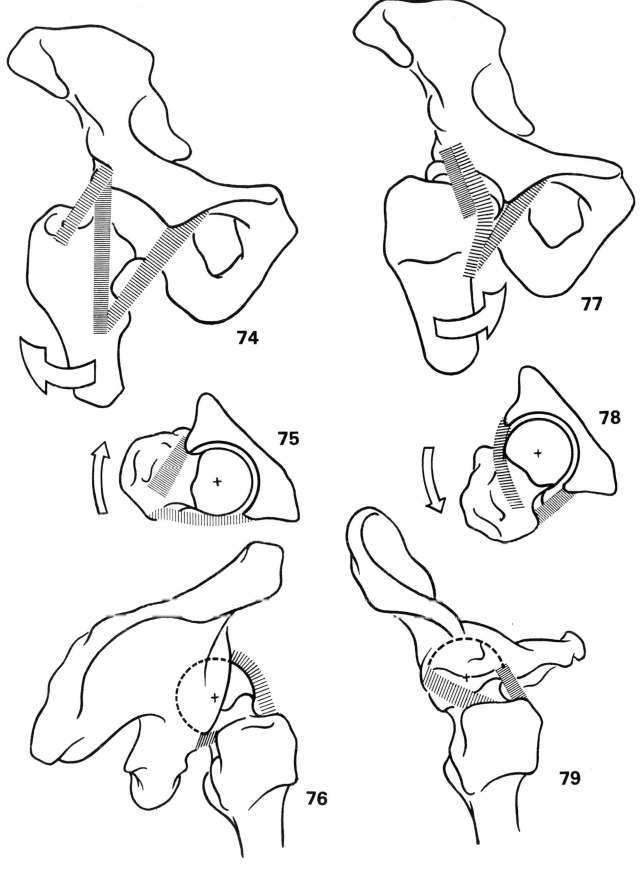

ROLE OF THE LIGAMENTS IN ADDUCTION AND ABDUCTION

Starting from the erect position (fig. 80), where the anterior ligaments are under moderate tension, it is clear that:

during adduction (fig. 81) the iliotrochanteric band becomes taut while the pubofemoral ligament is slackened. The inferior band is tightened only slightly;

during abduction (fig. 82) the opposite takes place: the pubofemoral ligaments are tightened considerably while the iliotrochanteric band and, to a lesser extent, the inferior band relax;

the **ischiofemoral ligament** (seen from behind) *is stretched during adduction* (fig. 83) and *tenses up during abduction* (fig. 84).

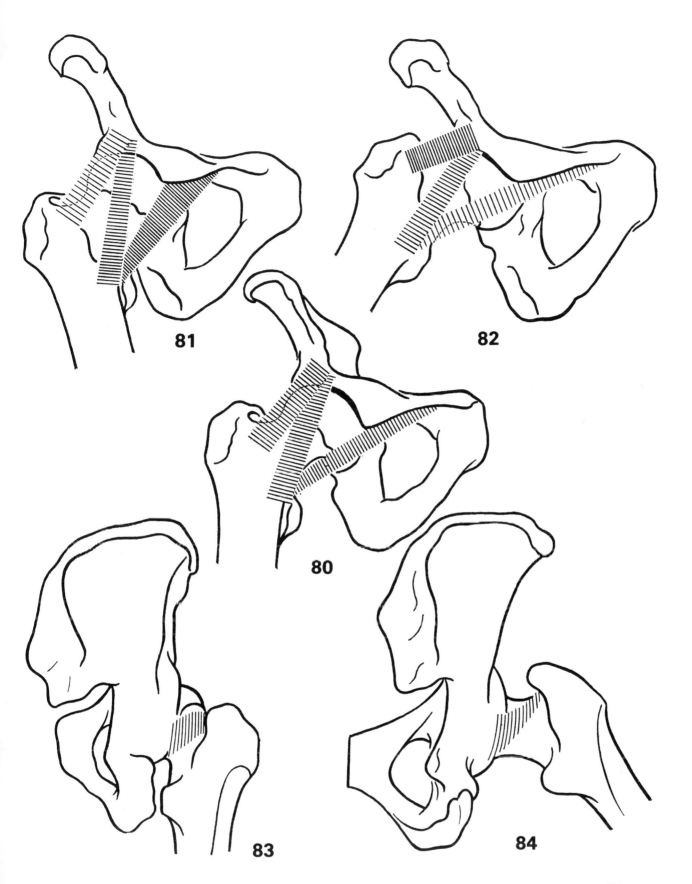

81

82

80

83

84

33

THE PHYSIOLOGICAL ACTIONS OF THE LIGAMENTUM TERES

This is an *anatomical vestige* and plays only a minor role in the control of the movements of the hip.

In **the erect position** (fig. 85: coronal section) it is under moderate tension and its femoral insertion lies in its intermediate position (1) in the acetabular fossa (fig. 86: diagram of the acetabular fossa showing the various positions of the fovea capitis femoris), i.e. slightly inferiorly and posteriorly to the centre (+).

During **flexion of the hip joint** (fig. 87) the ligament is twisted round itself and the fovea (fig. 86) comes to lie superior and anterior to the centre of the acetabular fossa (2). Hence the ligament plays no part in limiting flexion.

During **medial rotation** (fig. 88: horizontal section, seen from above) the fovea is displaced posteriorly and the femoral insertion of the ligament comes into contact with the posterior part of the articular crescent (3). The ligament remains moderately taut.

During **lateral rotation** (fig. 89) the fovea moves anteriorly and the ligament comes into contact with the anterior part of the articular crescent (4); here again the ligament is only moderately tensed. Note the impact of the posterior aspect of the femoral neck on the acetabular rim via the labrum, which becomes flattened and everted.

During **abduction** (fig. 90) the fovea moves inferiorly towards the acetabular notch (5) and the ligament is folded on itself. The labrum is squashed between the superior aspect of the neck and the acetabular margin.

During **adduction** (fig. 91) the fovea moves superiorly (6) to touch the roof of the acetabular fossa (6). This is the only position where the ligament is really under tension. The inferior border of the neck flattens slightly the labrum and the transverse ligament.

Therefore it becomes apparent that the acetabular fossa (including its posterior extension (7) and its anterior extension (8)) *encompasses all the various positions assumed by the foveal attachment of the ligamentum teres*. These two extensions correspond to the foveal position during adduction-extension-medial rotation (7), and adduction-flexion-lateral rotation (8). Between these two extensions of the fossa the articular cartilage shows a shallow indentation, which corresponds to the position of minimal adduction, i.e. in the frontal plane with the other limb checking adduction early. Therefore the inner outline of the articular cartilage is not due to chance but represents *the locus of the extreme positions of the foveal attachment of the ligamentum teres*.

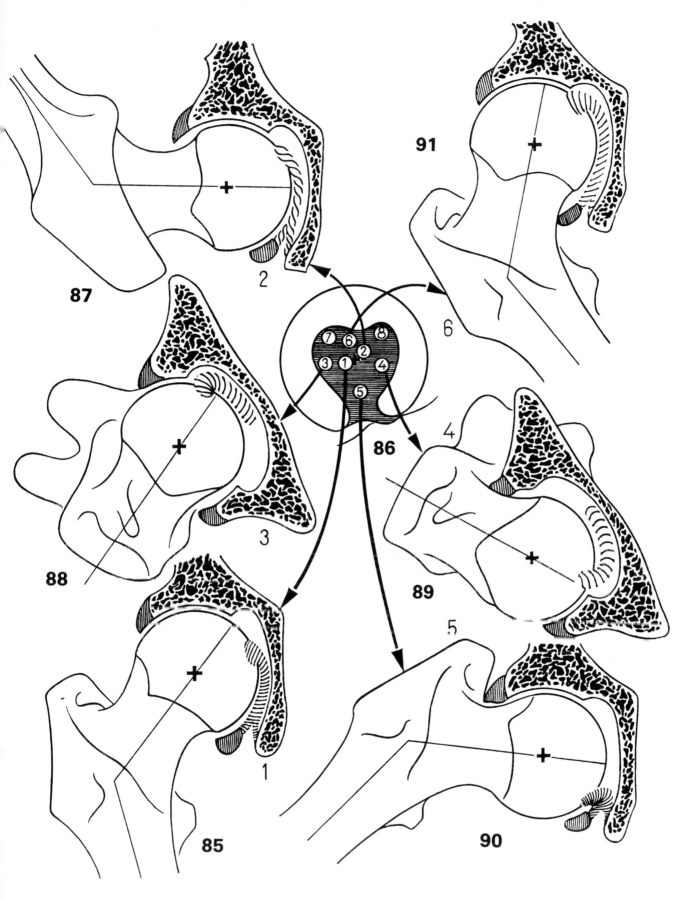

87

91

2

6

86

88

3

4

89

85

1

5

90

COAPTATION OF THE ARTICULAR SURFACES OF THE HIP

In contrast with the shoulder, which tends to be dislocated by the force of gravity, the hip is assisted by **gravity**, at least in the erect position (fig. 92). To the extent that the roof of the acetabulum covers the femoral head, the latter is pressed against the acetabulum by a force (ascending arrow) equal and opposition to the weight of the body (descending arrow).

It is known that the acetabulum is no more than a hemisphere. Therefore, in mechanical terms, there cannot be *true interlocking* of the surfaces since the femoral head cannot be retained mechanically by the hemispherical bony acetabulum. However, the **labrum acetabulare** widens and deepens the acetabulum so that the *acetabular cavity exceeds a hemisphere* (black arrows). Hence the hip is transformed into a proper ball-and-socket joint with *the fibrocartilaginous labrum holding the femoral head*. This fibrous interlocking is further enhanced by the **zona orbicularis** of the capsule which encircles the femoral head (shown in section by the small arrows).

Atmospheric pressure plays an important part in maintaining apposition of the articular surfaces, as proved by *the experiments of the Weber brothers*. They noted that, if all the soft tissue connections (including the capsule) were severed between the hip bone and the femur, the femoral head did not leave the acetabulum spontaneously and in fact could only be pulled away with great difficulty (fig. 93). If on the other hand (fig. 94) a small hole had been drilled into the depths of the acetabulum, the femur fell away under its own weight. If the hole was stopped after replacing the femoral head into the acetabulum, it was again very difficult to remove the head from the acetabulum. This experiment can be compared to the *classical experiment of Magdebourg*. He showed that it is impossible to separate two hemispheres after a vacuum has been created inside (fig. 95), whereas it is very easy to do so once air has been allowed in by a tap (fig. 96).

The **ligaments** and the **periarticular muscles** play a *vital part* in the maintenance of the structural integrity of the joint. Note (fig. 97: horizontal section) that their functions are reciprocally balanced. Thus anteriorly the muscles are very few (white arrow A) and the ligaments powerful while poseriorly the muscles (B) predominate.

Note also that the action of the ligaments varies *according to the position of the hip*: in the erect position or in extension (fig. 98) the ligaments are under tension and are efficient in securing coaptation; in flexion (fig. 99) the ligaments are relaxed (p. 28) and the femoral head is not as powerfully applied to the acetabulum. This mechanism can be understood easily from the mechanical model (fig. 100): parallel fibres run between two wooden circles (a) and, when one circle moves circularly relative to the other (b), the distance between them is reduced.

The *position of flexion* is therefore a *position of instability* because of the slackness of the ligaments. When a measure of adduction is added to the flexion, as in the sitting position with legs crossed (fig. 101), a relatively mild force applied along the femoral axis (arrow) is enough to cause posterior dislocation of the hip joint with or without fracture of the posterior margin of the acetabulum (e.g. impact on the dashboard during car accidents).

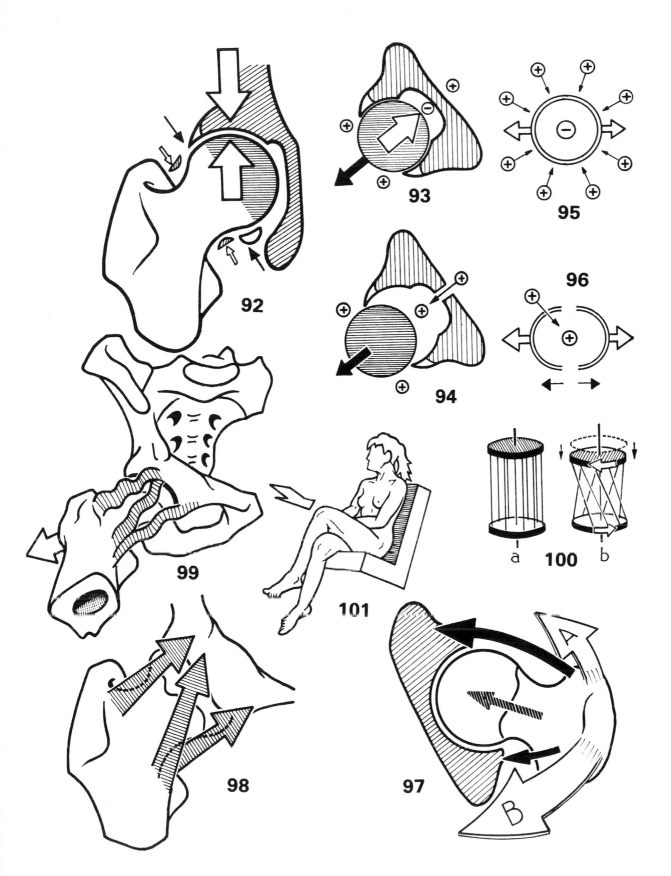

92

93

95

96

94

99

100

a   b

101

98

97

A

B

THE MUSCULAR AND BONY FACTORS INFLUENCING THE STABILITY OF THE HIP

The periarticular muscles are essential for the stability of the hip joint on condition, however, that they run transversely. In effect (fig. 102) *the muscles, running roughly parallel to the femoral neck,* keep the femoral head in contact with the acetabulum e.g. the pelvitrochanteric muscles—the piriformis (1) and the obturator externus (2) only shown here; the glutei, especially the minimus and the medius (3), which possess a powerful component of force (black arrow) producing coaptation. These muscles are therefore called the muscles of apposition of the hip. On the other hand, *longitudinal muscles,* like the adductors (4), tend to dislocate the femoral head above the acetabulum (right side, fig. 102), especially if the roof of the acetabulum is everted. This acetabular malformation is present in congenital dislocation of the hip and is easily recognised in an anteroposterior radiogram of the pelvis (fig. 103). Normally the angle of Hilgenreiner between the horizontal line running through the cartilages at level Y and the line running tangential to the acetabular roof is 25° in the neonate and 15° after the first year; when this angle exceeds 30° congenital malformation of the acetabulum is present. Dislocation is recognised by the upward displacement of the 'nucleus' of the head above the Y line (landmark of Putti) and the inversion of the angle of Wiberg (see fig. 36). In the presence of an acetabular malformation the adductors (4') can produce dislocation, the more so when the limb is adducted (fig. 102); on the other hand, the 'dislocating' component of the adductors decreases with increased abduction until in full abduction the adductors eventually favour apposition of the surfaces (fig. 104).

The **direction of the femoral neck** in both frontal and horizontal planes is of considerable importance in maintaining the stability of the joint. It has been shown (p. 14) that in the frontal plane the axis of the neck forms an angle of 120° to 125° with the axis of the shaft (fig. 105, a: diagram of the hip seen from in front). In congenital dislocation of the hip this angle can reach 140° (b) producing a coxa valga so that during adduction (c) the axis of the neck has already a 'head start' of 20° over its normal counterpart. Therefore a 30° adduction in a pathological hip (P) corresponds to a 50° adduction in a normal hip. Now adduction is known to enhance the dislocating action of the adductors. Hence **coxa valga promotes dislocation**. On the other hand, this abnormal hip will be stabilised in abduction; hence the use of the various positions of immobilisation for treatment of the congenital dislocation of the hip, the first being abduction at 90° (fig. 106).

In the horizontal plane (fig. 107: diagram of the hip seen from above) the angle between the axis of the femoral neck and the frontal plane has a mean value of 20° (a). Because the axes of the femoral neck and of the acetabulum are out of line in the erect posture (p. 16), the anterior part of the femoral head lies outside the acetabulum. If this angle is increased to, say, 40° (b) and the femoral neck runs more anteriorly, this is called *anteversion of the femoral neck* and the head is more liable to anterior dislocation. In fact, for a lateral rotation of 25° (c) the axis of a normal neck falls within the acetabulum (N) whereas the axis of an anteverted neck (P), which already has a 20° 'headstart', will fall on the acetabular rim so that the head is liable to anterior dislocation. Therefore **anteversion of the femoral neck favours dislocation of the joint**. Conversely, retroversion of the neck promotes stability in the same way as medial rotation (d). This is why the third position of reduction of congenital dislocation of the hip combines the 'straight' position and *medial rotation* (fig. 106).

These architectural and muscular factors are extremely important in maintaining the **stability of a prosthesis**. Thus during total hip replacement the surgeon must secure the following:

the proper orientation of the neck without excessive anteversion, while using the anterior approach and vice versa.

the proper orientation of the prosthetic acetabulum, which, like the original acetabulum, must face inferiorly with an angle less than 45°–50° to the horizontal and slightly anteriorly with an angle less than 15°.

the restoration of the 'functional length' of the femoral neck by ensuring the normality of the lever arm of the gluteal muscles which are essential for the stability of a prosthesis.

Emphasis must also be placed on the choice of the surgical approach with minimal disruption of the periarticular muscles.

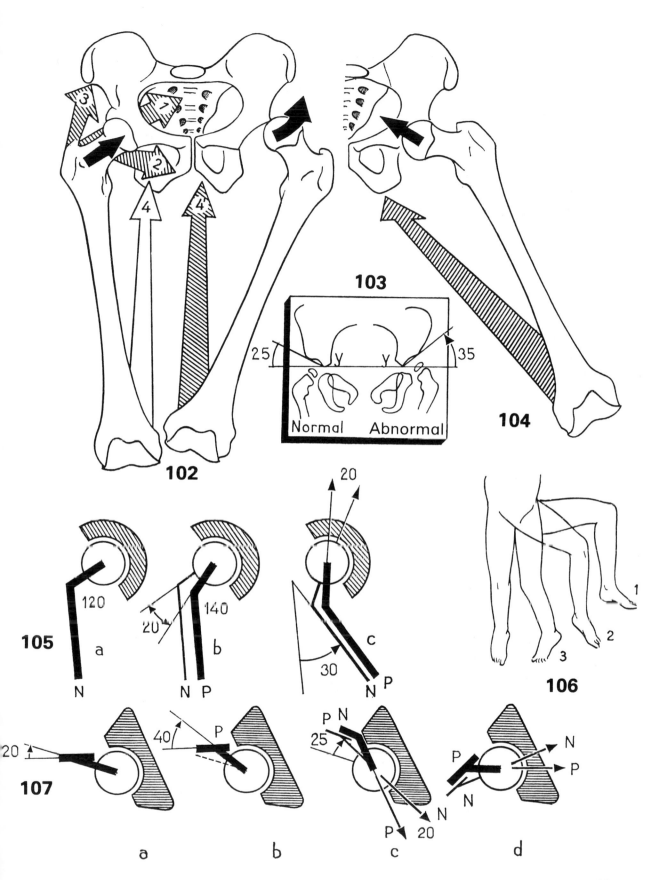

102

103

25 y y 35

Normal   Abnormal

104

105

120

a

20 140

b

20

30

c

N   N P   N P

106

1

2

3

107

20

a

40 P

b

P N

25

20

P N

N

c

P

N

P

N

d

39

THE FLEXOR MUSCLES OF THE HIP

These muscles lie *anterior to the frontal plane, which passes through the centre of the joint* (fig. 108). They all run *anterior to the axis of flexion and extension* XX' lying in this frontal plane.

There are many flexor muscles of the hip and the most important are the following (fig. 109):

The **psoas** (1) and the **iliacus** (2) share a common tendon of insertion into the lesser trochanter; this tendon bends sharply at the level of the iliopubic eminence. The iliopsoas muscle is the most powerful of the flexors and has the longest range (the highest fibres of the psoas being inserted into the twelfth thoracic vertebra). Its action as an adductor is challenged by many authors in spite of its course medial to the anteroposterior axis. This lack of any adductor action could be due to the fact that the apex of the lesser trochanter lies on the mechanical axis of the lower limb (fig. 48). However, in support of its adductor action, one notes that on the skeleton the lesser trochanter is nearest to the iliopubic eminence during flexion-adduction-lateral rotation. The iliopsoas also produces lateral rotation.

The **sartorius** (3) is mainly a flexor of the hip and secondarily produces abduction and lateral rotation (fig. 110); it also acts on the knee (flexion and medial rotation: p. 142). It is fairly powerful (muscular pull equivalent to 2 kg. weight) and nine-tenths of its power is expended in flexion.

The **rectus femoris** (4) is a powerful flexor (equivalent to 5 kg. weight) but its action on the hip depends on the degree of flexion of the knee. It is more efficient the more the knee is flexed (p. 000). It is particularly so in movements combining knee extension and hip flexion, as when the limb moves forward during walking (fig. 111).

The **tensor fasciae latae** (5) is a fairly powerful flexor in addition to being a stabiliser of the pelvis and an abductor of the hip (p. 48).

Some muscles are only *accessor flexors* of the hip but their contribution to flexion is not negligible:

the **pectineus** (6) which is primarily an adductor;

the **adductor longus** (7), primarily adductor but also partially flexor (p. 58);

the **gracilis** (8);

the most anteior fibres of the glutei, minimus and medius (9).

All these flexors of the hip can produce adduction/abduction or lateral/medial rotation as accessory movements and they can be divided into two groups according to these actions:

The *first group* includes the anterior fibres of the glutei, minimus and medius (9) and the tensor fasciae latae (5). They produce flexion-abduction-medial rotation (right thigh, fig. 109) and they are involved alone or predominantly in the production of the footballer's movement shown in figure 112.

The *second group* includes the iliopsoas (1 and 2), pectineus (6) and the adductor longus (7) which produce flexion-adduction-lateral rotation (left thigh, fig. 109); this complex movement is illustrated in figure 113.

During simple flexion, as in walking (fig. 111), these two groups must act as a *balanced set of synergists and antagonists*. In flexion-adduction-medial rotation (fig. 114) the adductors and the tensor fasciae latae play a dominant role, assisted by the medial rotators, the glutei minimus and medius.

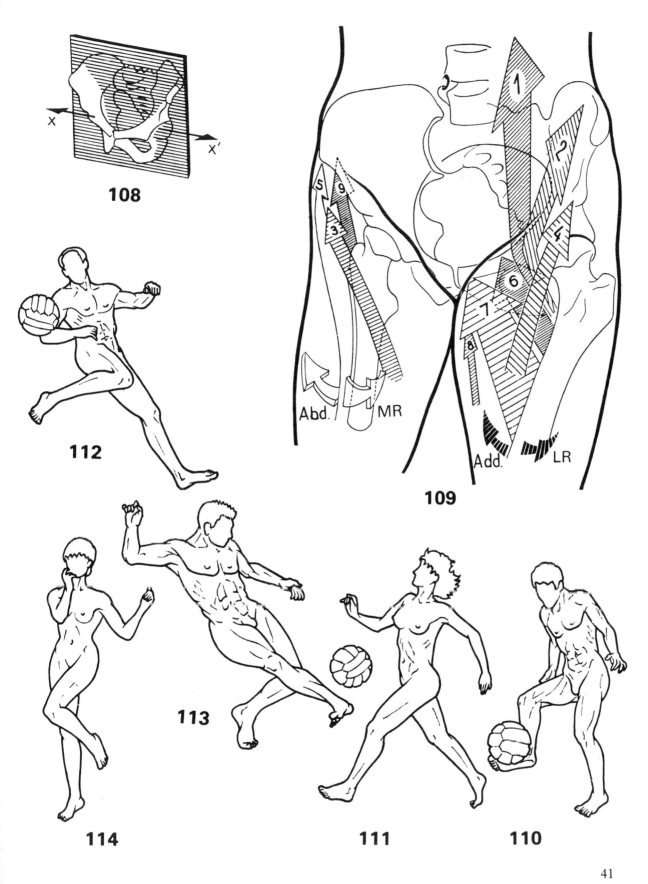

108

112

109

Abd.   MR

Add.   LR

113

114   **111**   **110**

41

THE EXTENSOR MUSCLES OF THE HIP

These muscles *lie posterior to the frontal plane that passes through the centre of the joint* (fig. 115) and contains the transverse axis XX' of flexion and extension.

There are **two main groups of muscles**: the one group is inserted into the femur and the other in the vicinity of the knee joint (fig. 116).

Of the *first group* the **gluteus maximus** (1 and 1') is the most important. It is the most powerful muscle of the body (force equivalent to 34 kg. weight; contraction length of muscle = 15 cm.), and is also the biggest (66 cm.^{2} in cross-section) and, naturally, the strongest (its static power is equivalent to 238 kg. weight). It is assisted by the *most posterior fibres of the glutei, medius (2) and minimus (3)*. These muscles are also lateral rotators (p. 54).

The *second group* consists essentially of the **hamstring muscles** i.e. biceps femoris (4), semitendinosus (5), seminembranosus (6); their power is equivalent to 22 kg. weight i.e. two-thirds that of the gluteus maximus. They are biarticular muscles and *their efficiency at the hip depends on the position of the knee*: the locking of the knee in extension enhances their extensor action at the hip; this suggests a synergism between the hamstrings and the quadriceps femoris (especially the rectus). This group also includes some adductors, especially the adductor magnus (7) which is an *accessory* extensor of the hip (see page 52).

The extensor muscles of the hip have *secondary actions* depending on their position relative to the anteroposterior axis YY' of adduction and abduction:

those running *superior to the axis YY'* produce abduction along with the extension as in the dancing movement shown in figure 117. These muscles include the most posterior fibres of the glutei, minimus (3) and medius (2) and the most superior fibres of the gluteus maximus (1');

those running *inferior to the axis YY'* produce abduction and extension as in the movement shown in fig. 118. These muscles are the hamstrings, the adductors (i.e. those lying behind the frontal plane) and the bulk of the gluteus maximus (1).

To produce pure extension (fig. 119) i.e. without associated adduction and abduction, these two muscle groups are thrown into balanced contraction as synergists and antagonists.

The extensors of the hip joint play an essential part in *stabilising the pelvis in the anteroposterior direction* (fig. 120):

When the pelvis is tilted posteriorly (a), i.e. in the direction of extension, it is stabilised only by the tension of the iliofemoral ligament (IFL) which limits extension (p. 28); there is a position (b) where the centre of gravity (c) of the pelvis lies directly above the centre of the hip. The flexors and extensors are not active but the equilibrium is unstable; when the pelvis is tilted anteriorly (c) the centre of gravity (c) comes to lie in front of the transverse axis of the hips and the hamstrings (H) are the first to contract so as to straighten the pelvis; when the pelvis is tilted very far anteriorly (d) the gluteus (G) maximus contracts powerfully as well as the hamstrings, which are more efficient the greater the degree of knee extension (standing with trunk bent forwards and the hands touching the feet).

During normal walking extension is produced by the hamstrings and *the gluteus maximus is not involved*. However, when one is running, jumping or walking up a slope, the gluteus maximus is essential and plays an important part.

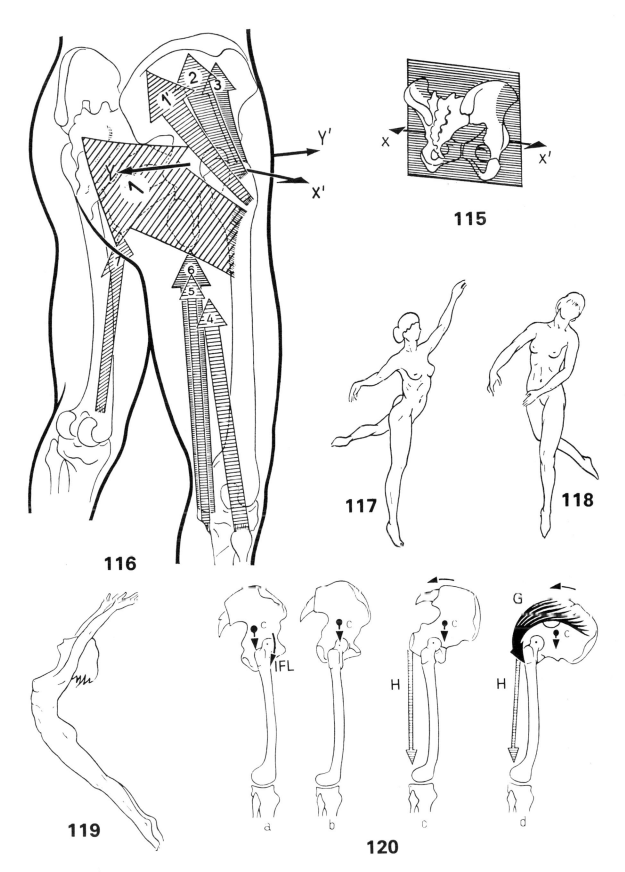

115

116

117

118

119

120

THE ABDUCTOR MUSCLES OF THE HIP

These muscles **generally lie lateral to the sagittal plane which traverses the centre of the joint** (fig. 121) and run laterally and superiorly to the **anteroposterior axis YY' of adduction and abduction** contained in that sagittal plane.

The main abductor muscle is the **gluteus medius** (1). It has a cross-sectional area of 40 cm.^{2} and it contracts by 11 cm. It can produce a force equivalent to 16 kg. weight. It is highly efficient because it is almost perpendicular to its lever arm OT (fig. 122). It is also essential, along with the gluteus minimus, for the stabilisation of the pelvis in the transverse direction (p. 48).

The **gluteus minimus** (2) is essentially an abductor (fig. 123).

It has a cross-sectional area of 15 cm.^{2} and it shortens by 9 cm. during contraction. It can produce a force equivalent to 5 kg. weight, i.e. about one-third that of the gluteus medius.

The **tensor fasciae latae** (3) is a powerful abductor of the hip when it is in the erect position. Its muscular power is about half of that of the gluteus medius (7.6 kg weight) but its lever arm is much longer than that of the gluteus medius. It also acts to stabilise the pelvis.

The **gluteus maximus** (4) produces abduction only with its highest fibres (the bulk of the muscle produces adduction) and its superficial fibres, which form part of the so-called 'deltoid of the hip' (fig. 127).

The **piriformis** (5) is undoubtedly an abductor but its action cannot be easily demonstrated experimentally because of its deep location.

According to their secondary movements of flexion/extension and adduction/abduction, these abductor muscles can be classified into two groups:

The first group includes all the muscles lying anterior to the frontal plane running through the centre of the joint, i.e. tensor fasciae latae, the anterior fibres of the gluteus medius, and the bulk of the gluteus minimus. These muscles, whether they contract alone or are assisted by weaker fellows, produce **abduction-flexion-medial rotation** (fig. 124).

The *second group* consists of the posterior fibres of the glutei, minimus and medius (the fibres lying posterior to the frontal plane) and the abductor fibres of gluteus maximus. These muscles, whether they contract alone or are assisted by weaker fellows, produce **abduction-extension-lateral rotation** (fig. 125).

To obtain **pure abduction** (fig. 126), i.e. without any other associated movements, these two groups of muscles must be activated as a balanced couple of synergists-antagonists.

44

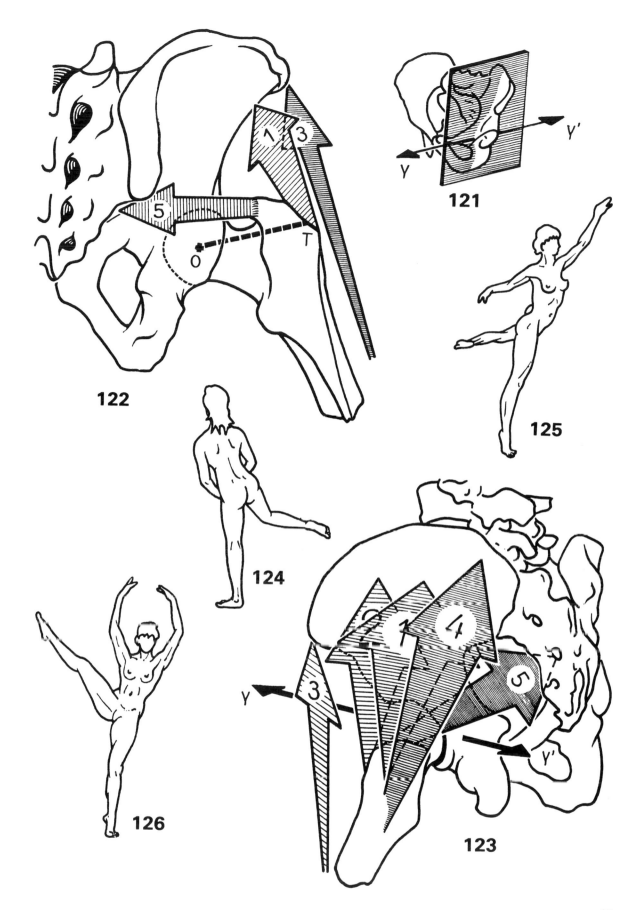

121

122

124

125

126

123

45

THE TRANSVERSE STABILITY OF THE PELVIS

When the **pelvis is supported on both sides** (fig. 131), its stability in the transverse direction is secured by the simultaneous contraction of the ipsilateral and contralateral adductors and abductors. When these antagonistic actions are properly balanced (a) the pelvis is stabilised in the position of symmetry, as in the military position of standing to attention. If the abductors predominate on one side and the adductors on the other (b), the pelvis is tilted laterally towards the side of adductor predominance. If muscular equilibrium cannot be restored at this point the subject will fall to that side.

When the **pelvis is supported by only one limb** (fig. 132), the stability of the pelvis is provided solely by the action of the ipsilateral abductors, since the weight of the body P, acting through the centre of gravity, will tend to tilt the pelvis at the supporting hip. The pelvis can therefore be compared to a lever system of type I (fig. 133), where the fulcrum is the supporting hip O, the disturbing force is the weight of the body P acting through the centre of gravity G and the restoring force is the muscular pull of gluteus medius (GMe) acting at the external iliac fossa E. To keep the pelvis horizontal when supported on one leg, the muscular force of gluteus medius must cancel the force exerted by the body weight, taking into account that the lever arms OE and OG are not equal in length. In this action the gluteus medius is powerfully assisted by gluteus minimus and the tensor fasciae latae (fig. 132).

If there is insufficiency of any one of these muscles (fig. 132, b) the body weight acting at G is not properly counterbalanced and the pelvis tilts to the opposite side to form an angle α with the horizontal, which is directly proportional to the severity of the muscular insufficiency. The tensor fasciae latae stabilises not only the pelvis but also the knee: therefore (p. 106) it is effectively an **active** collateral ligament so that its paralysis in the long run leads to an abnormal widening of the knee joint interspace laterally (angle β).

Stabilisation of the pelvis by the glutei and the tensor fasciae latae is essential for normal walking (fig. 134). While the pelvis is supported on one limb, the transverse axis of the pelvis, represented by the interiliac line, stays horizontal and parallel to the line joining the two shoulders. If these muscles are paralysed on the side supporting the pelvis (fig. 135), the pelvis is tilted to the opposite side. This would result in a fall to that side, if the whole trunk were not bent towards the supporting side and the line of the shoulders tilted the same way. This combination of movements during walking—i.e. tilting of the pelvis towards the unsupported side and bending of the upper trunk towards the supported side—is very characteristic and is used clinically (sign of Duchenne-Trendelenburg) to demonstrate complete or partial paralysis of the glutei, minimus and medius.

48

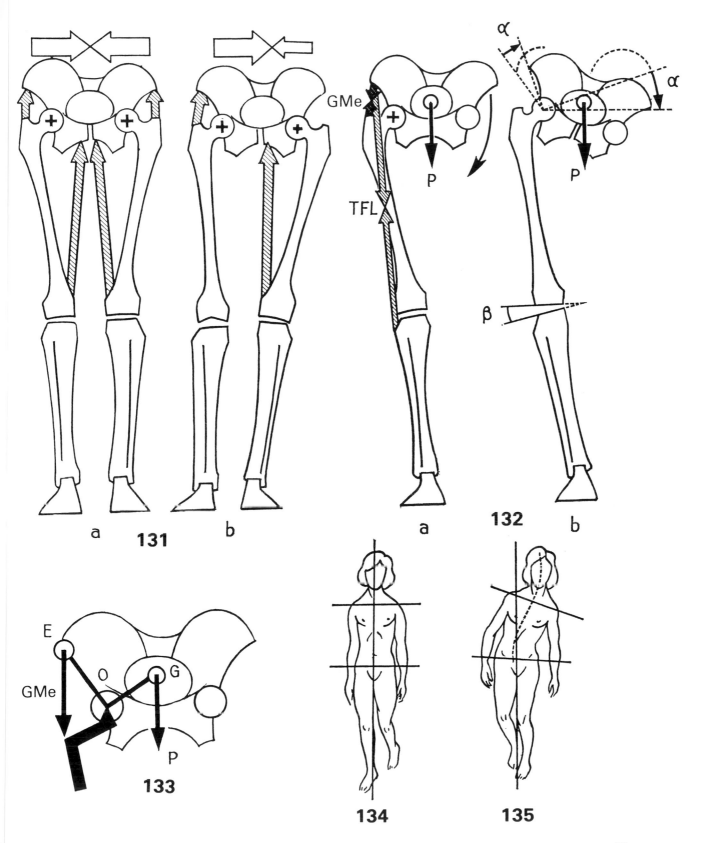

a   131   b

a   132   b

GMe

TFL

P

P

α

α

β

E

GMe

O   G

P

133

134   135

49

THE ADDUCTOR MUSCLES OF THE HIP—*(Continued)*

The adductor muscles are seen from the front in figure 140:

the **adductor longus** (13) whose muscular power (equivalent to 5 kg. weight) falls short of half that of the adductor magnus;

the **adductor brevis** (14): its two bundles are covered inferiorly by the adductor longus and superiorly by the pectineus;

the **gracilis** (4) which forms the internal border of the adductor compartment.

In addition to their primary adductor action the muscles also produce some measure of flexion-extension and axial rotation.

Their role in flexion and extension (fig. 141: seen from inside) depends upon the site of their origin. If they arise from the hip bone *posterior* to the frontal plane which runs through the centre of the joint (line of alternate dashes and dots), they produce extension, especially the inferior fibres of the adductor magnus (i.e. the 'third adductor') and, of course, the hamstrings. If the muscles arise from the hip bone *anterior* to that frontal plane, they produce flexion, e.g. pectineus, adductor brevis and adductor longus, upper fibres of the adductor magnus and gracilis. Note, however, that their role in flexion and extension depends also on the initial position of the hip (p. 58).

The adductors, as shown previously, are essential for the stabilisation of the pelvis when supported on both limbs; they therefore play an essential part in certain postures or movements in sport e.g. skiing (fig. 142) and horse-riding (fig. 143).

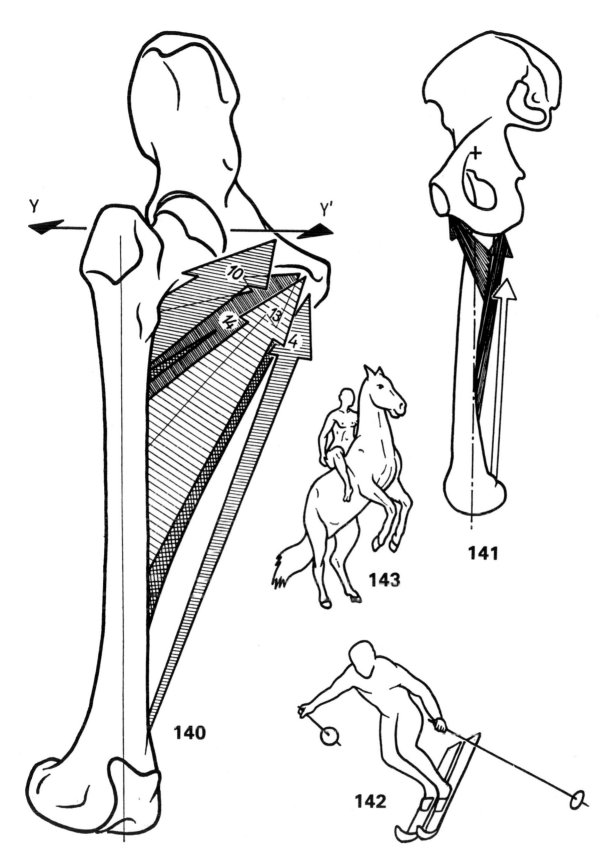

140

141

143

142

THE LATERAL ROTATOR MUSCLES OF THE HIP

These are **numerous** and **powerful**. *During their course they cross the vertical axis of the hip posteriorly,* as is shown by a *horizontal section* of the pelvis passing slightly above the centre of the joint (fig. 144: seen from above). This diagram shows all the lateral rotators, which are:

the **pelvitrochanteric muscles** with lateral rotation as primary function:

the **piriformis** (1), arising from the inner surface of the sacrum, runs anteriorly and laterally, emerges through the greater sciatic foramen (fig. 145: seen from behind and above) and is inserted by tendon into the superior margin of the greater trochanter;

the **obturator internus** (2) arises from the side wall of the pelvis around the obturator foramen and runs part of its course within the pelvic cavity (2'). At the level of the lesser sciatic foramen its tendon bends sharply at right angles (fig. 145), emerges through the lesser sciatic foramen and runs parallel to the piriformis to its insertion into the medial surface of the greater trochanter. Outside the pelvis the muscle is accompanied by the **two gemelli**, which are two tiny muscles arising respectively from the margins of the lesser sciatic notch. They run along the superior and inferior borders of the obturator internus and are inserted via its tendon into the greater trochanter. They have a similar action;

the **obturator externus** (3) arises from the external surface of the margins of the obturator foramen and its tendon winds posteriorly below the hip joint and runs upwards behind the femoral neck to its insertion into the floor of the trochanteric fossa. On the whole the muscle winds its way round the femoral neck and can only be seen in its entirety when the pelvis is considerably tilted on the femur (fig. 146: postero-infero-lateral view of the pelvis with the hip flexed). This explains its two main actions: it is especially a lateral rotator when the hip is flexed (p. 56) and is slightly flexor because of its winding course round the femoral neck.

Some adductor muscles are also lateral rotators:

the **quadratus femoris** (4) arising from the ischial tuberosity and inserted into the trochanteric crest and quadrate tubercle (fig. 145). It can also extend or flex the hip according to the position of the latter (fig. 153);

the **pectineus** (6) arising from the pectineal border and surface of the pubis and inserted into the femur along the line joining the lesser trochanter and the linea aspera (fig. 146). It produces adduction, flexion and lateral rotation;

the most posterior fibres of the adductor magnus also produce lateral rotation like the hamstrings (fig. 147);

the **glutei**:

the **gluteus maximus** as a whole is a lateral rotator, including its superficial (7) and deep (7') fibres;

the posterior fibres of the gluteus minimus and especially of the **gluteus medius** (8) (figs. 144 and 145).

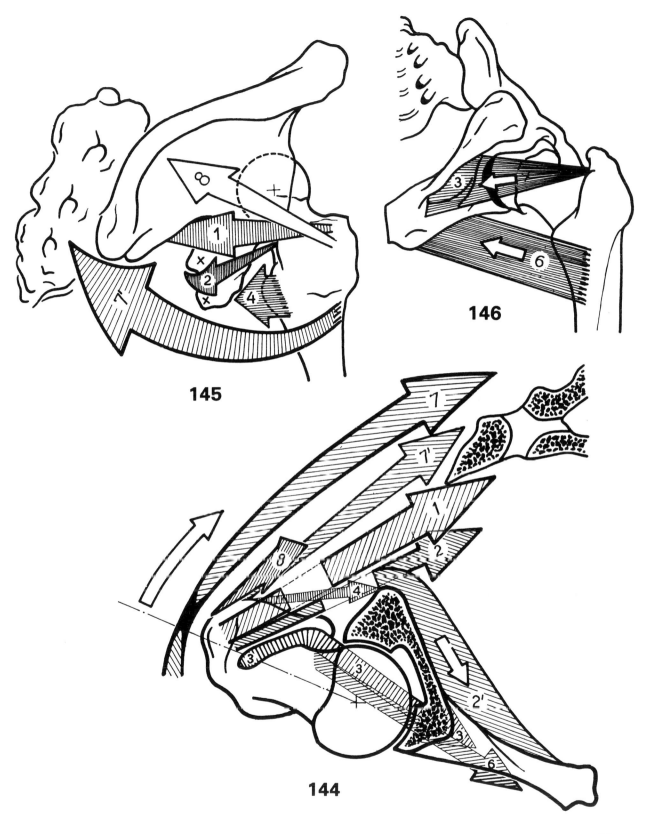

145

146

144

INVERSION OF MUSCULAR ACTION

The motor muscles of a joint with three degrees of freedom do not have the same action whatever the position of the joint; their secondary actions can be altered and even reversed. The most typical example is **the inversion of the flexor component of the adductor muscles** (fig. 152). Starting from the erect position (0°) all the adductors are flexors except the posterior fibres of the adductor magnus and especially the 'third adductor' (TA), which is and remains extensor right up to −20° extension. But this flexor component operates only so long as the femur still lies inferior to the site of origin of each muscle. So the adductor longus (AL) is still flexor at position +50° but becomes extensor at +70°. Likewise the adductor brevis is flexor up to +50°, after which it produces extension. For the gracilis the limit of flexor action is +40°. The diagram shows that only the true flexors can produce flexion right up to the limit. At +120° the tensor fasciae latae (TFL) is shortened maximally (i.e. by a length aa′ equal to half the length of its muscle fibres), while the psoas (P) has almost run out of useful contraction since its tendon now tends to 'take off' from the iliopectineal eminence. (The diagram suggests an explanation of 'why' the lesser trochanter is situated very far posteriorly: the excursion of the psoas tendon is thereby increased by a length equal to the thickness of the femoral shaft.)

The **quadratus femoris** also shows this inversion of muscular action very clearly (fig. 153: the transparent iliac bone allows the femur and the quadratus to be seen): in extension (E) of the hip the quadratus is flexor, while in flexion it becomes extensor; the point of transition corresponds to the erect position of the hip.

The **efficiency of the muscles** depends largely on *the position of the hip*. When the joint is already flexed (fig. 154) the extensor muscles are under tension. With flexion of 120° the gluteus maximus is passively lengthened by a length GG′, which for certain fibres represents 100 per cent. lengthening; the hamstrings are lengthened (HH′) by about 50 per cent. of their length in the 'straight' position of the hip provided the knee stays extended. This explains the starting position of runners (fig. 155): maximal flexion of the hip followed by extension of the knee (this second phase is not illustrated), which produces the right amount of tension in the hip extensors for the powerful movement of the start. It is this tension of the hamstrings that checks flexion of the hip when the knee is extended.

Figure 154 also shows that from the erect position to that of extension at −20° the change in length of the hamstrings (HH″) is relatively small. This confirms the idea that the hamstrings work at their best advantage when the hip is half-flexed.

58

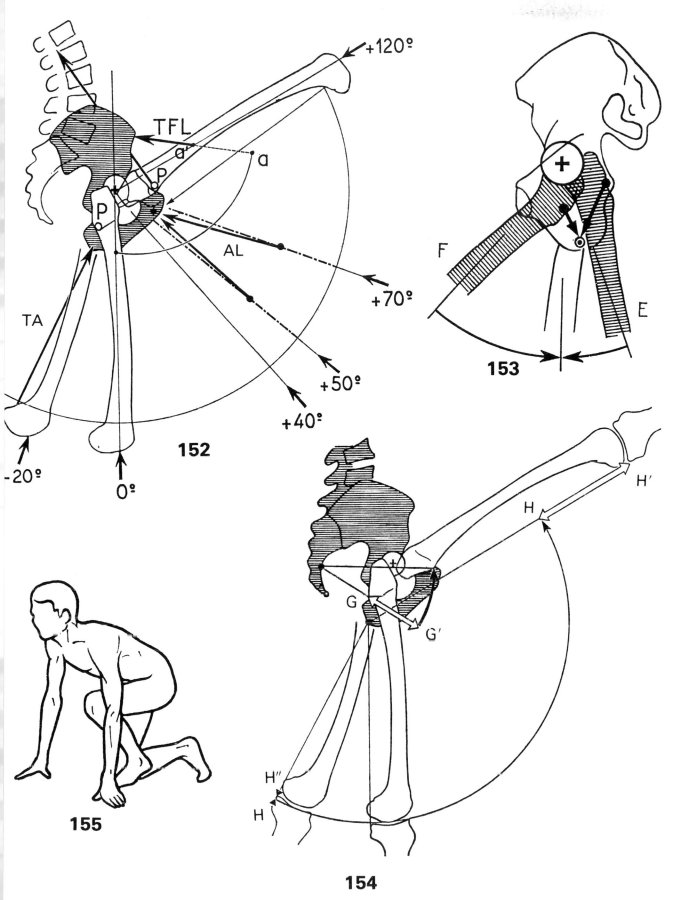

152

TFL

a'

a

P

P

AL

TA

+120°

+70°

+50°

+40°

-20°

0°

153

F

E

+

154

G

G'

H

H'

H

H"

+

155

59

SUCCESSIVE RECRUITMENT OF THE ABDUCTOR MUSCLES

Depending on the degree of flexion of the hip, the pelvis, **when supported on one limb**, is stabilised by different abductor muscles.

When the hip is extended (fig. 161), the centre of gravity of the body falls posterior to the transverse axis of the two hips. The posterior tilting of the pelvis is checked by the tension of the iliofemoral ligament (p. 28) and contraction of the tensor fasciae latae which is also a flexor of the hip. Hence the tensor fasciae latae corrects simultaneously posterior and lateral tilting of the pelvis.

If the pelvis is only slightly tilted posteriorly (fig. 162) the centre of gravity still lies posterior to the axis of the hips and the gluteus minimus is thrown into action. Note that this muscle also produces abduction with flexion like the tensor fasciae latae.

When the pelvis is in equilibrium in the anteroposterior plane (fig. 163) the centre of gravity lies on the axis of the hips and the pelvis is laterally stabilised by the gluteus medius.

When the pelvis is tilted forward the gluteus maximus is called into action and subsequently the piriformis (fig. 164), the obturator internus (fig. 165) and the quadratus femoris (fig. 166), are recruited as flexion of the trunk increases. These muscles are also *abductors* (when the hip is flexed) and *extensors*, so that they can compensate for any tilt of the pelvis in the anteroposterior and transverse planes.

62

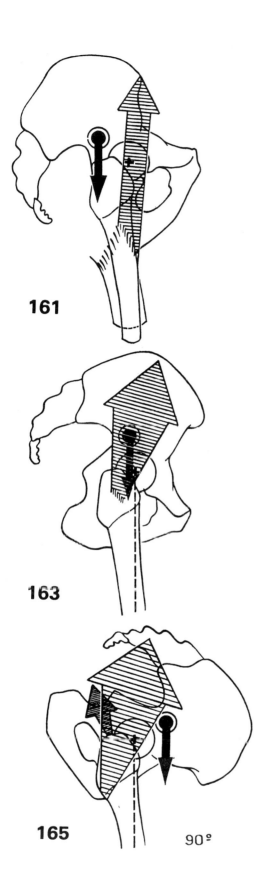

161

162

163

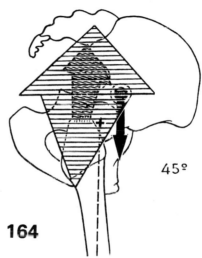

164

45°

165

90°

166

110°

The Knee

The knee is the *intermediate* joint of the lower limb. It is *mainly* a joint with **one degree of freedom** which allows the end of the limb to be moved towards or away from its root or, in other words, allows the distance between the trunk and the ground to be varied. *The knee works essentially by axial compression* under the action of gravity.

The knee has an **accessory, i.e. second, degree of freedom**: rotation of the long axis of the leg, which only occurs *when the knee is flexed*.

From the mechanical point of view the knee is a compromise which sets out to reconcile **two mutually exclusive requirements**:

to have *great stability* in complete extension, when the knee in subjected to severe stresses resulting from the body weight and the length of the lever arms involved;

to have *great mobility* after a certain measure of flexion has been achieved. This mobility is essential for running and the optimal orientation of the foot relative to the irregularities of the ground.

The knee resolves this problem by highly ingenious mechanical devices but the poor degree of interlocking of the surfaces—essential for great mobility—renders it liable to sprains and dislocations.

During **flexion** the knee is unstable and the ligaments and menisci are most susceptible to injury.

During **extension**, injury to the knee is most likely to result in fractures of the articular surfaces and rupture of the ligaments.

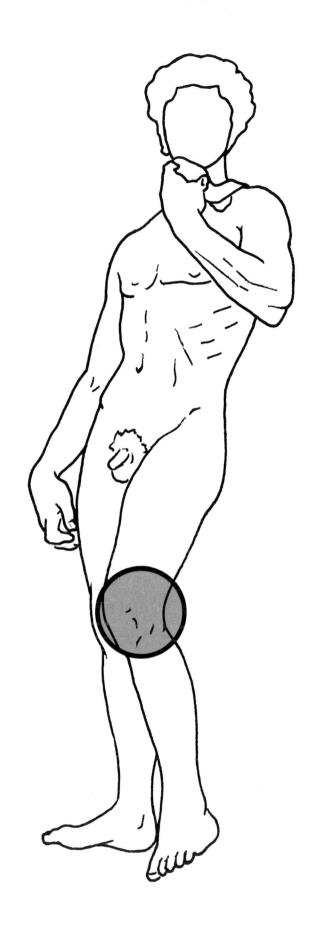

65

THE AXES OF THE KNEE

The **first degree of freedom** is related to the *transverse axis* XX' (fig. 1, semiflxed knee seen from inside; fig. 2, seen from outside), around which occur movements of flexion and extension in a sagittal plane. This axis XX', lying in a frontal plane, runs through the femoral condyles horizontally.

Because the femoral neck overhangs the shaft (fig. 3), the axis of the femoral shaft does not coincide with that of the leg but forms with the latter an obtuse angle of 170 to 175° opening outwards. This is the *physiological valgus of the knee.*

On the other hand, the centres of the three joints, i.e. hip (H), knee (O), ankle (C), lie on a straight line HOC which is the **mechanical axis** of the lower limb. In the leg it coincides with that of the leg itself but in the thigh it forms an acute angle of 6° with the axis of the femur.

Because the hips are wider apart than the ankles, *the mechanical axis of the lower limb runs obliquely inferiorly and medially* and forms an angle of 3° with the vertical. This angle is greater the wider the pelvis, as in the case of women. This also explains why the physiological valgus of the knee is *more marked in women* than in men.

The axis of flexion and extension XX' is horizontal and so does not coincide with Ob which bisects the angle of valgus. The angle between XX' and the femoral axis is 81° and that between XX' and the axis of the leg is 93°. Therefore during full flexion the axis of the leg does not come to rest immediately posterior to that of the femur but *posterior and slightly medial to it* so that the heel moves medially towards the plane of symmetry of the body. Full flexion brings *the heel into contact with the buttock at the level of the ischial tuberosity.*

The second degree of freedom of the joint is related to rotation around the *long axis* YY' of the leg (figs. 1 and 2) *with the knee flexed.* The structure of the knee makes **axial rotation impossible when the knee is fully extended**; the axis of the leg coincides with the mechanical axis of the lower limb and axial rotation occurs not at the knee but at the hip, which is thus complementary to the knee.

In figure 1 an axis ZZ' (broken line) is shown running anteroposteriorly and at right angles to the other two axes. This axis does not represent a third degree of freedom but, owing to a measure of 'play' at the joint, **side-to-side movements** occur (1 to 2 cm. when measured at the ankle). In full extension these movements disappear and if they still persist they must be considered, as a rule, as *abnormal.*

It must be remembered that *transverse displacements occur normally during flexion.* To determine whether these displacements are normal or abnormal they **must be compared with those of the other knee**, provided that the latter is normal.

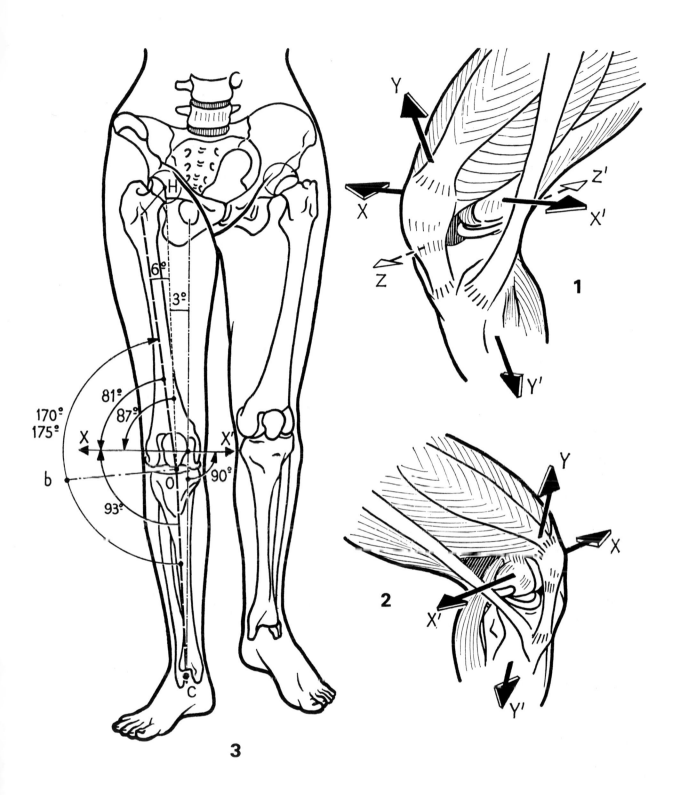

1

2

3

MEDIAL AND LATERAL DISPLACEMENTS OF THE KNEE

In addition to its sex-related physiological range, **the degree of valgus shows individual pathological variations** (fig. 4).

Inversion of the angle of valgus produces the *genu varum* (fig. 4: left side), i.e. **bandy legs** (fig. 6). The centre of the joint, running through the tibial interspinal groove and the femoral intercondylar fossa, is displaced **laterally**. **Genu varum** can be quantitated *in two ways*:

by **measuring the angle** between the femoral and tibial shafts. It then *exceeds* its normal value of 170°, e.g. 180°–185°, with inversion of the obtuse angle between the shafts.

by **measuring the lateral displacement** (fig. 5) of the centre of the joint with respect to the mechanical axis of the lower limb, e.g. 10–20 mm.

Conversely, closure of the valgus angle gives rise to the **genu valgum** (fig. 4: right side), i.e. **knock knees** (fig. 8). Here again there are *two ways* of quantitating the deformity:

by **measuring the angle** between the femoral and tibial shafts, which is less than the normal value of 170°, e.g. 165°.

by **measuring the medial displacement** (fig. 7) of the centre of the joint with respect to the mechanical axis of the lower limb, e.g. 10–20 mm.

Measurement of **transverse displacements** is more precise than measurement of the angle of valgus but it requires **comprehensive radiographs or the lower limb of sufficient quality to allow accurate measurements** (fig. 4) **or gonometry.** In the diagram, by bad luck, the patient has a right genu valgum and a left genu varum. This occurrence is rare, as in most cases the deformity is similar on both sides but not necessarily symmetrical in terms of severity. There are, however, very rare cases where the displacements of the centre of the joint take place in the same direction. This combined deformity is very uncomfortable with loss of stability of the genu valgum. It can arise when an osteotomy has overcorrected a genu varum or a genu valgum. It is then imperative to operate on the other knee without delay to restore normal balance.

Transverse displacements of the knee are not harmless as they can cause osteoarthritis. In fact, mechanical loads are unevenly spread over the two compartments of the knee joint with premature erosion of the medial or lateral compartment, i.e. **medial or lateral femoro-tibial osteoarthritis**, in genu varum or valgum respectively. Treatment may then necessitate the appropriate form of tibial or femoral osteotomy.

It is precisely to prevent these complications that a lot of attention is now being paid to transverse displacements of the knee in young children. It is a fact that bilateral genu valgum is very common in children and disappears with growth. Nevertheless, this favourable outcome should be followed with comprehensive radiographs of the lower limb. If a significant displacement were to persist at the end of childhood, the need might arise for medial or lateral arthrodesis for genu valgum or varum respectively. Surgery should be performed before the end of the growth period as these operations work by inhibiting the growth of one side of the knee with respect to the other.

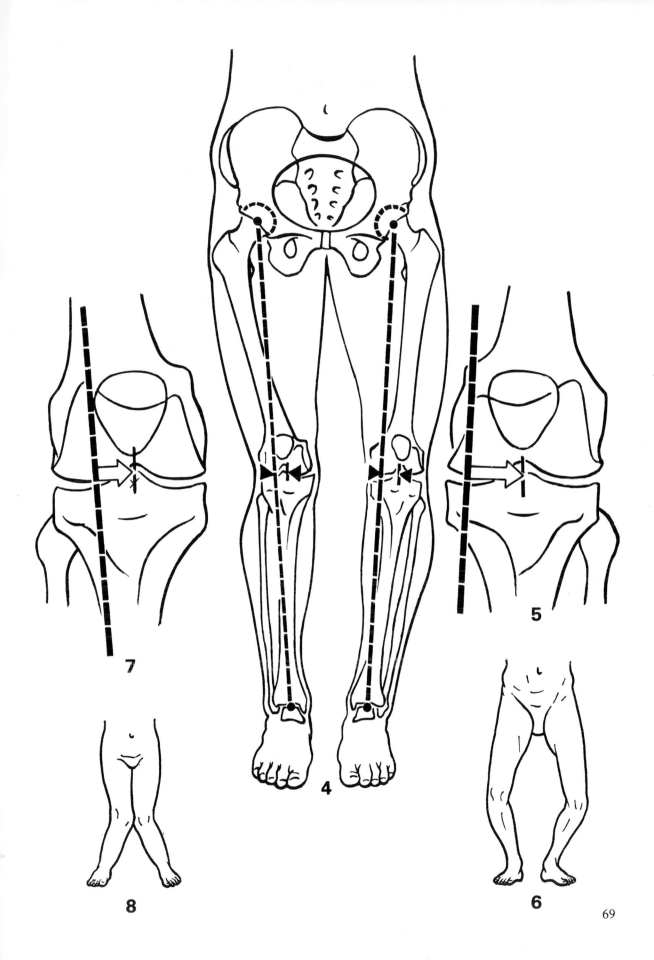

7

4

8

5

6

MOVEMENTS OF FLEXION AND EXTENSION

These are the main movements of the knee and their range is measured from the **position of reference** established by the following criterion: *the axis of the leg is in line with that of the thigh* (fig. 9, left leg), i.e. seen from the side, the axis of the femur prolongs that of the leg directly. In this position of reference, the lower limb is at its longest.

Extension is defined as the movement of the posterior aspect of the leg *away* from the posterior surface of the thigh. There is strictly no **absolute extension** since in the position of reference the limb is maximally extended. It is, however, possible to achieve *passive extension* (5° to 10°) from the position of reference (fig. 11): this is wrongly called 'hyperextension'. In some people this hyperextension can be abnormally marked leading to the *genu recurvatum*.

Active extension goes beyond the position of reference rarely and then only slightly (fig. 9) and this depends upon the position of the hip joint. In fact, the efficiency of the rectus femoris as an extensor of the knee increases with extension of the hip (p. 138), so that extension of the hip (fig. 10: right leg) sets the stage for kneee extension.

Relative extension is the movement which brings the knee into full extension starting from any position of flexion (fig. 10: left leg). It occurs normally during walking when the limb off the ground is extended to resume contact with the ground.

Flexion is the movement of the posterior aspect of the leg *towards* the posterior aspect of the thigh. Flexion can be *absolute*, i.e. from the reference position, and *relative*, i.e. from any position of partial flexion.

The range of knee flexion varies according to the position of the hip and according to whether it is active or passive.

Active flexion attains a range of 140° if the hip is already flexed (fig. 12) and only 120° if the hip is extended (fig. 13). This difference is due to the fact that the hamstrings lose some of their efficiency with extension of the hip (p. 140). It is, however, possible to exceed 120° flexion with the hip extended as a result of a '*follow-through*' *effect*. When the hamstrings contract abruptly and powerfully the knee is thrown into flexion and the end of active flexion is followed by a measure of passive flexion.

Passive flexion of the knee attains a range of 160° (fig. 14) and *allows the heel to touch the buttock*. This movement underlies an important clinical test of the freedom of flexion of the knee and the range of passive flexion of the knee can be assessed in terms of the distance between the heel and the buttock. Normally, flexion is checked only by the apposition of the elastic muscle masses of the calf and the thigh. Pathologically, passive flexion is checked only by the apposition of the elastic muscle masses of the calf and the thigh. Pathologically, passive flexion is limited by *retraction of the extensor apparatus*—essentially the quadriceps—or by *shortening of the capsular ligaments* (p. 98).

It is possible to quantitate a **flexion deficit** by either computing the difference between the degree of flexion achieved and the maximum expected (160°) or by measuring the distance between the heel and the buttock. In contrast, an **extension deficit** is reckoned as a **negative angle**, i.e. −60°, lying between the position attained by passive extension and the neutral position. Thus in figure 13 it can be said that the leg is flexed at 120° or, if it cannot be further extended, that it displays an **extension deficit of −120°**.

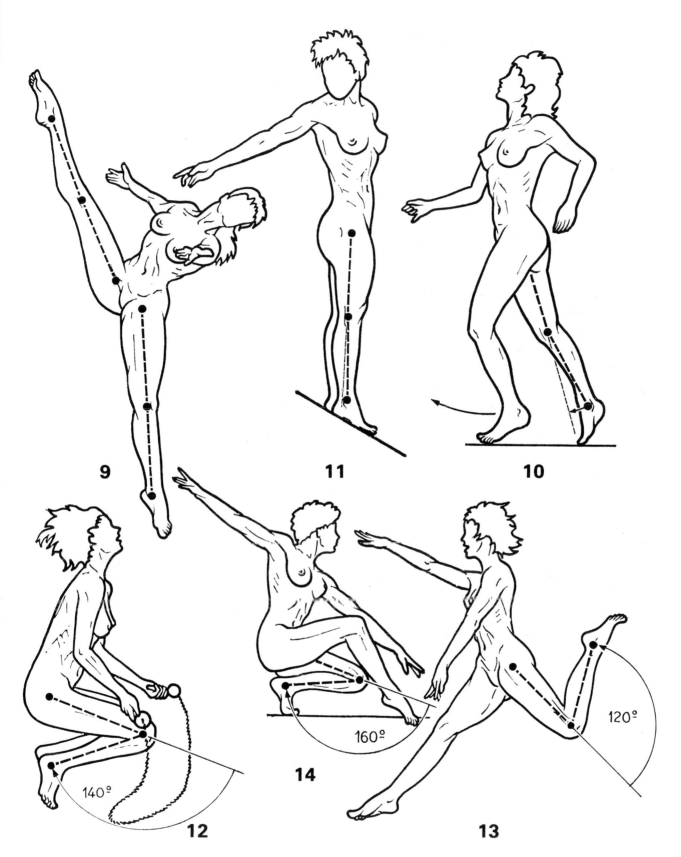

9

11

10

12 140°

14 160°

13 120°

71

AXIAL ROTATION OF THE KNEE

Rotation of the leg around its long axis can only be performed with the knee flexed.

To measure **active axial rotation** the knee must be flexed at right angles with the subject sitting at the edge of a table with his legs hanging down (fig. 15); knee flexion prevents rotation at the hip. In the position of reference the toes face slightly outwards (p. 74).

Medial rotation (fig. 16) brings the toes to face *medially* and plays an important part in adduction of the foot (p. 168).

Lateral rotation (fig. 19) brings the toes to face *laterally* and also plays an important part in abduction of the foot.

According to Fick, lateral rotation has a range of 40° and medial rotation a range of 30°. This range varies with the degree of knee flexion since, according to the same author, lateral rotation attains a 32° range when the knee is flexed at 30° and 42° range when the knee is flexed at right angles.

Passive axial rotation can be measured when the subject lies prone with the knee flexed. The examiner grasps the foot with both hands and turns it so that the toes face outwards (fig. 18) and inwards (fig. 19). As expected, this passive rotation has a greater range than active rotation.

Finally there is also a type of **axial rotation called automatic** because it is inevitably and involuntarily linked to movements of flexion and extension. It occurs especially at the end of extension or the start of flexion. When the knee is extended the foot is *laterally (EXTernally) rotated* (fig. 20); hence the mnemonic EXTension and EXTernal rotation. Conversely, when the knee is flexed the leg is *medially rotated* (fig. 21). The same movement takes place when one tucks the lower limbs underneath the trunk and the toes are brought to face medially (the foetal position).

The mechanism of this automatic axial rotation will be discussed later.

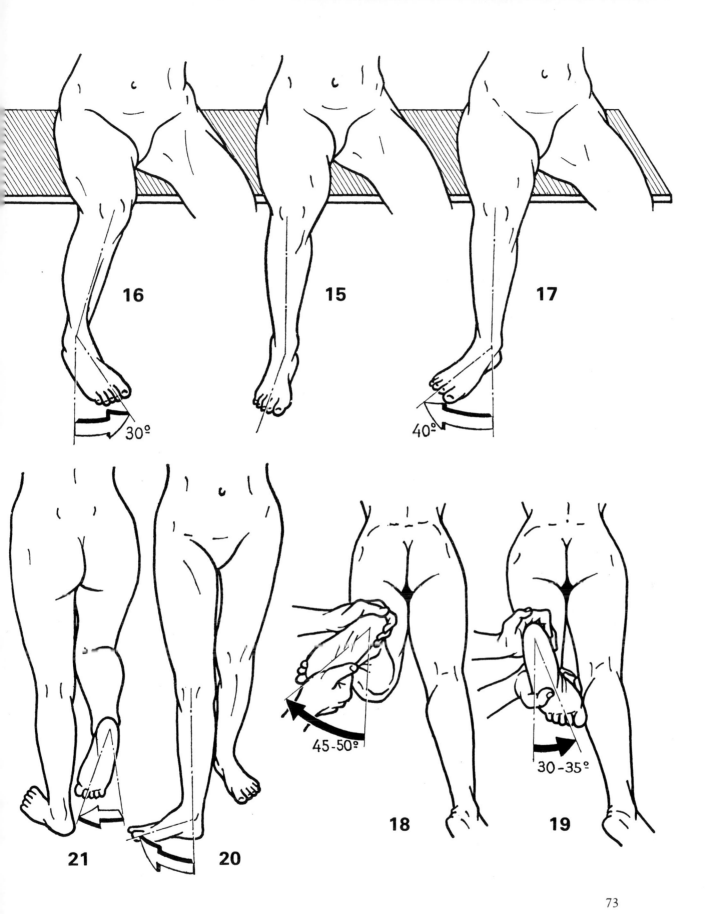

16

15

17

30°

40°

21

20

18

19

45-50°

30-35°

THE GENERAL STRUCTURE OF THE LOWER LIMB AND ORIENTATION OF THE ARTICULAR SURFACES

The orientation of the femoral condyles and the tibial condyles favours flexion of the knee (fig. 22, according to Bellugue). Two bony extremities, moving relative to each other (a), become moulded according to their movements (b) (experiment of Fick, Vol. III). Flexion falls short of a right angle (c) unless a small fragment (d) is removed from the upper bone so as to delay contact of the two bones. The weak point thus created in the bone is compensated by forward displacement (e) of the shaft so that the condyles come to lie posteriorly. Reciprocally, the tibia is thinned posteriorly and reinforced anteriorly (f) so that the tibial plateau comes to lie more posteriorly. Thus, during extreme flexion, large muscular masses can be lodged between tibia and femur.

The overall curvatures of the lower limb reflect the stresses which are applied and obey the laws of Euler governing the behaviour of *columns eccentrically loaded* (Steindler). If a column is jointed at its two ends (fig. 23a) the bend involves the whole length of the column; hence the bend of the femur, concave posteriorly (fig. 23b). If the column is fixed below and mobile above (fig. 24a) two bends with opposite curvatures are seen, with the higher bend taking up two-thirds of the column; these bends correspond to those of the femur in the frontal plane. If the column is fixed at both ends (fig. 25a) the bend takes up its two middle fourths; this corresponds to the bends of the tibia in the frontal plane (fig. 25b). In the sagittal plane the tibia shows the following three features (fig. 26b):

retrotorsion (T), i.e. posterior displacement of the upper end, already mentioned;

retroversion (V), i.e. the tibial condyles are inclined posteriorly at an angle of 5° to 6° with the horizontal;

retroflexion (F), i.e. the tibia is bent so as to be concave posteriorly; this corresponds to the bend seen in a column which is mobile at both ends (fig. 26a), as with the femur.

During flexion (fig. 27) the concavities of the femur and tibia face each other and so increase the space for lodgement of the soft tissue masses.

The diagrams at the bottom of the page constitute a sort of 'anatomical algebra', attempting to explain *the successive movements of axial torsion of the bones of the lower limb*, as seen from above.

Torsion of the femur (fig. 28): let us assume that (a) the head and neck (1) and the condyles (2) constitute a single solid structure. If no torsion is present (b) the axis of the neck lies in the same plane as that of the condyles. However, in life, the neck forms an angle of 30° with the frontal plane (c): therefore, if the axis of the condyles is to stay in the frontal plane (d), the *femoral shaft must be twisted by* −30° *of medial rotation*.

Torsion of the tibia (fig. 29): let us assume (a) that the ankle (1) and the tibial condyles (2) form one solid structure. In the absence of any torsion (b) the axis of the condyles and that of the ankle lie in a frontal plane. But in life (c) the retroposition of the external malleolus causes the axis of the ankle to run obliquely laterally and posteriorly; this corresponds to a *torsion of the tibia equivalent to* +25° *of lateral rotation*.

Let us now consider (fig. 30a) the femoral (1) and the tibial (2) condyles together. It looks as if their two axes should lie in a frontal plane (b). In life, *automatic axial rotation* produces +5° of lateral rotation of the tibia on the femur during full extension of the knee.

These torsions, staggered over the whole length of the lower limb (−30° +25° +5°), cancel out (fig. 31a) so that the axis of the ankle is roughly parallel to that of the femoral neck, i.e. showing 30° lateral rotation. Hence *the axis of the foot is set at* 30° *to the plane of symmetry* when one stands erect with heels together and the pelvis symmetrically balanced (b). During walking the movement of the advancing limb brings the ipsilateral hip forwards (c); if the pelvis turns by 30°, the axis of the foot comes to lie in a sagittal plane i.e. in the plane of movement and this allows the step to evolve under the best conditions.

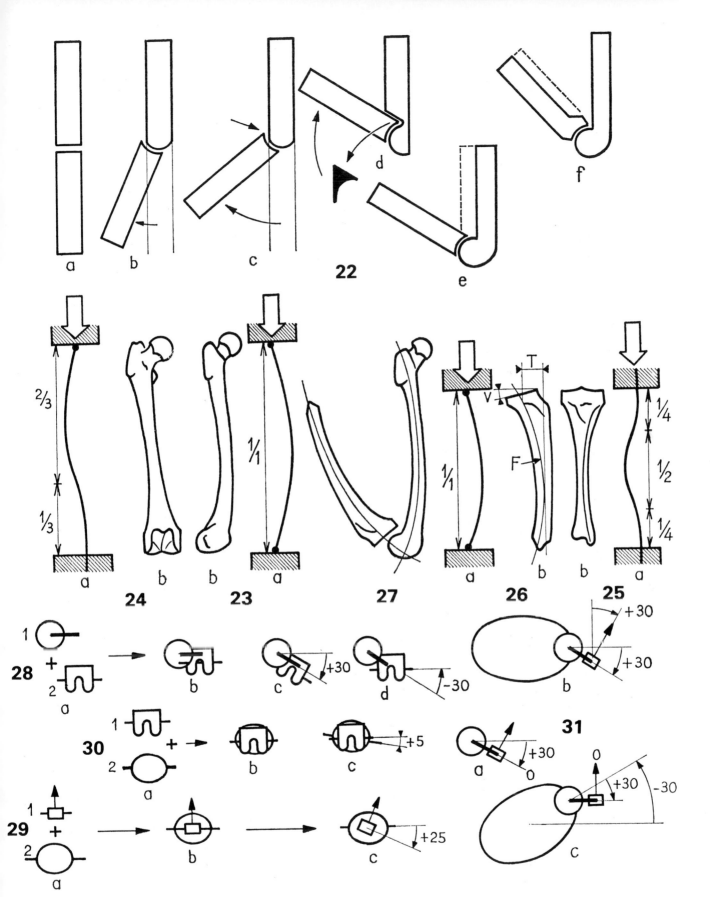

ARTICULAR SURFACES INVOLVED IN FLEXION AND EXTENSION

The main movement of the knee, i.e. flexion and extension, occurring around a transverse axis, depends upon the fact that it is a **hinge joint**. In fact, the articular surfaces of the femur are *pulley-shaped*, or, more exactly, represent a segment of a pulley (fig. 32), which recalls, in a general way, the *twin undercarriage of an aeroplane* (fig. 33). The two femoral condyles, convex in both planes, form the two lips of the pulley and correspond to the wheels of the aeroplane; they are extended anteriorly (fig. 34) by the pulley-shaped patellar surface. The neck of the pulley is represented anteriorly by the central groove on the patellar surface and posteriorly by the intercondylar notch (the mechanical significance of this arrangement will emerge later). Some authors describe the knee as a bicondyloid joint: this is true anatomically but from the mechanical point of view the joint is indisputably of the hinge variety.

The tibial surfaces are reciprocally curved and comprise *two curved and concave parallel gutters which are separated by a blunt eminence running anteroposteriorly* (fig. 35). The lateral condyle (LC) and the medial condyle (MC) lie each in a gutter on the surface S and are separated by a blunt anteroposterior eminence which lodges the two intercondylar tubercles. Anteriorly, if this eminence is prolonged, it coincides with the vertical ridge on the deep surface of the patella (P), while the two facets on either side of the patellar ridge correspond to the tibial condyles. These surfaces have a transverse axis (I) which coincides with the intercondylar axis (II) when the joint is closed.

Therefore the tibial condyles correspond to the femoral condyles while the intercondylar tibial tubercles come to lie within the femoral intercondylar notch: these surfaces constitute functionally **the femorotibial joint**. Anteriorly the two facets of the patella correspond to the patellar surface of the femur while the vertical ridge of the patella fits into the central groove of the femur: these surfaces constitute the second *functional* joint, i.e. the **femoropatellar joint**. These two functional joints are contained within a single anatomical joint, i.e. the knee.

From the point of view of flexion and extension, one can in the first instance consider the knee as made up of a pulley-shaped surface gliding in a twin set of curved and concave gutters (fig. 36). But, as will become obvious later, the situation is more complex in reality.

76

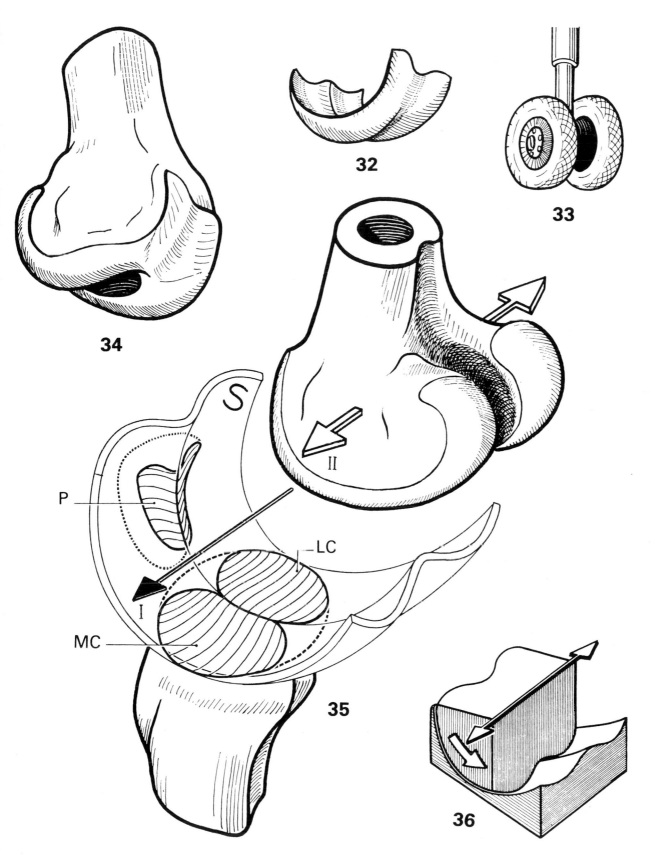

32

33

34

35

S

P

LC

I

MC

II

36

ARTICULAR SURFACES IN RELATION TO AXIAL ROTATION

As described on the preceding page, the articular surfaces allow only one movement, i.e. flexion and extension. In fact, the tibial intercondylar eminence by lodging in the intercondylar notch of the femur *along its whole length* would preclude any axial rotation of the tibia on the femur.

Hence, to allow axial rotation, the tibial surface (fig. 37) must be so modified as to shorten the intercondylar eminence. This is achieved by planing (fig. 38) the two ends of the eminence and leaving its middle part to act as a *pivot*, which, by lodging in the intercondylar notch, allows the tibia to rotate round it. This pivot consists of the **intercondylar spines** which form respectively the lateral border of the medial condyle and the medial border of the lateral condyle. The vertical axis (R), about which occur the movements of axial rotation, passes through this central pivot or more correctly through the medial intercondylar spine. Some authors give the label of central pivot to the cruciate ligaments, taken as the axis of rotation of the knee. This terminology is inappropriate since a pivot implies the presence of a *solid fulcrum*, which is best provided by the medial intercondylar spine. For the cruciate ligaments the term *central link* seems more suitable.

This modification of the articular surfaces is more easily understood with the help of a **mechanical model**.

Let us take two structures (fig. 39): the one above containing a *groove* and the one below a *shoulder*. Since the groove and the shoulder fit exactly, the two structures can *slide* one over the other but they *cannot turn* relative to each other.

If the two ends of the shoulder are removed leaving intact its central part which is rounded off so that its greatest diameter fits the groove (fig. 40), the shoulder is now replaced by a *cylindrical knob*, which can still fit into the groove of the upper surface.

Now (fig. 41) these two structures can undergo *two types of movement* relative to each other:

a sliding movement of the central knob along the groove corresponding to flexion/extension;

a movement of rotation of the knob inside the groove (whatever its location within the groove), corresponding to rotation around the long axis of the leg.

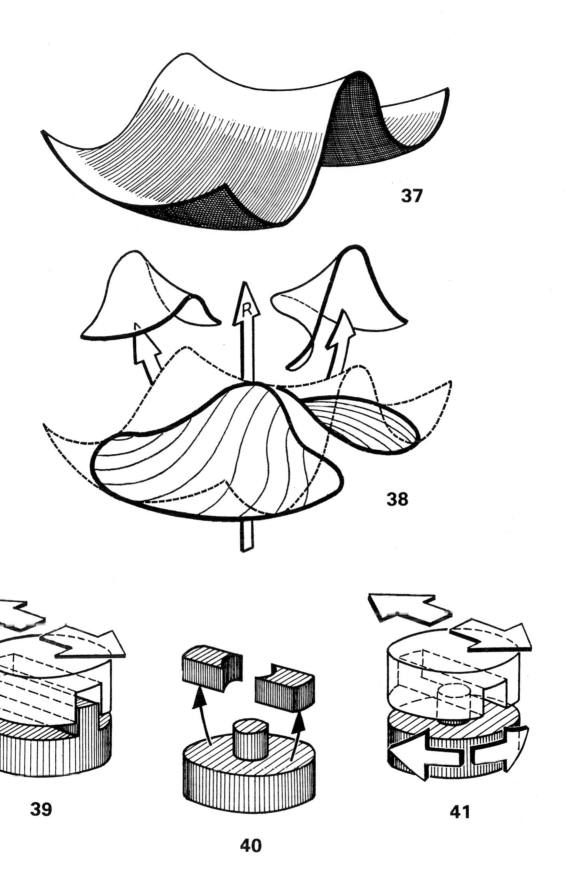

37

38

39

40

41

79

PROFILE OF THE FEMORAL AND TIBIAL CONDYLES

When seen from below (fig. 42) the **femoral condyles** form two prominences *convex in both planes* and longer anteroposteriorly than transversely. They are not strictly identical: their long axes (i.e. anteroposterior) are not parallel but *diverge posteriorly*. Moreover, the medial condyle (M) juts out far more than the lateral condyle (L) and is also narrower. Between the patellar surface of the femur and the condyles run the medial and lateral grooves (r), the medial one being more obvious than the lateral.

The **intercondylar notch** (e) lies on the axis of the *central groove of the patellar surface* (g). The lateral facet of this surface is *more prominent* than the medial facet.

The frontal section (fig. 43) shows that the convexity of the femoral condyles in the transverse plane corresponds to the concavity of the tibial condyles.

To study the **curvature of the femoral and tibial condyles** in the sagittal plane it is convenient to examine sagittal sections taken at the levels aa' and bb' (fig. 43). These sections taken from a fresh bone provided a faithful profile of the femoral and tibial condyles (figs. 45 to 48). It is then clear that the radius of curvature of the femoral condyles is not uniform but varies as in the case of a **spiral**.

In geometry, Archimedes' spiral (fig. 44) is constructed around a point called its centre C so that every time the radius R sweeps over an angle its length is correspondingly increased.

The **spiral of the femoral condyles** is *quite different*, though their radii of curvature increase regularly postero-anteriorly, i.e. from 17 to 38 mm. for the medial condyle (fig. 45) and from 12 to 60 mm. for the lateral condyle (fig. 46). But the spiral does not have only one centre but *a series of centres lying on a spiral mm'* (medial condyle) and nn' (lateral condyle). Therefore the curve of the condyles represents a *spiral of a spiral* as shown by Fick, who gave the name of **evolving curve** to this spiral.

On the other hand, starting from a **certain point t** on the edge of the condyle, the radius of curvature begins to decrease, i.e. from 38 to 15 mm. postero-anteriorly for the medial condyle (fig. 45) and from 60 to 16 mm. for the lateral condyle (fig. 46). Here too the centres of curvature lie on a spiral m'm" (medial condyle) and n'n" (lateral condyle). On the whole, *the lines joining these centres of curvature constitute two spirals lying back to back* and having a very sharp apex (m' and n'), which corresponds to the point t on the condyle, i.e. the point of transition between *the two segments of the condylar profile*:

posterior to point t, the part of the condyle belonging to the *femorotibial joint*;

anterior to point t, the part of the condyle and patellar surface of the femur belonging to the *femoropatellar joint*.

The transition point t represents the most extreme point of the condyle able to come into contact with the tibia.

We have demonstrated by a mechanical model that the trochleo-condylar profile is geometrically determined by the knee ligaments.

The **anteroposterior profile of the tibial condyles** (figs. 47 and 48) varies with the condyle examined.

the medial condyle (fig. 47) is *concave superiorly* (the centre of curvature O lies above) with a radius of curvature of 80 mm;

the lateral condyle (fig. 48) is *convex superiorly* (the centre of curvature O' lies below) with a radius of curvature of 70 mm.

Therefore, *while the medial condyle is biconcave, the lateral condyle is concave in the frontal plane and convex in the sagittal plane* (as seen in the fresh specimen). As a result, the medial femoral condyle is relatively stable inside the concave medial tibial condyle, while the lateral femoral condyle is unstable as it rides on the convex surface of the lateral tibial condyle. Its stability during movements depends on the integrity of the anterior cruciate ligament.

Also, the radii of curvature of the corresponding femoral and tibial condyles are not equal so that the articular surfaces are not congruent. In fact *the knee typifies joints with incongruent surfaces*. The restoration of congruence rests with the menisci (p. 92).

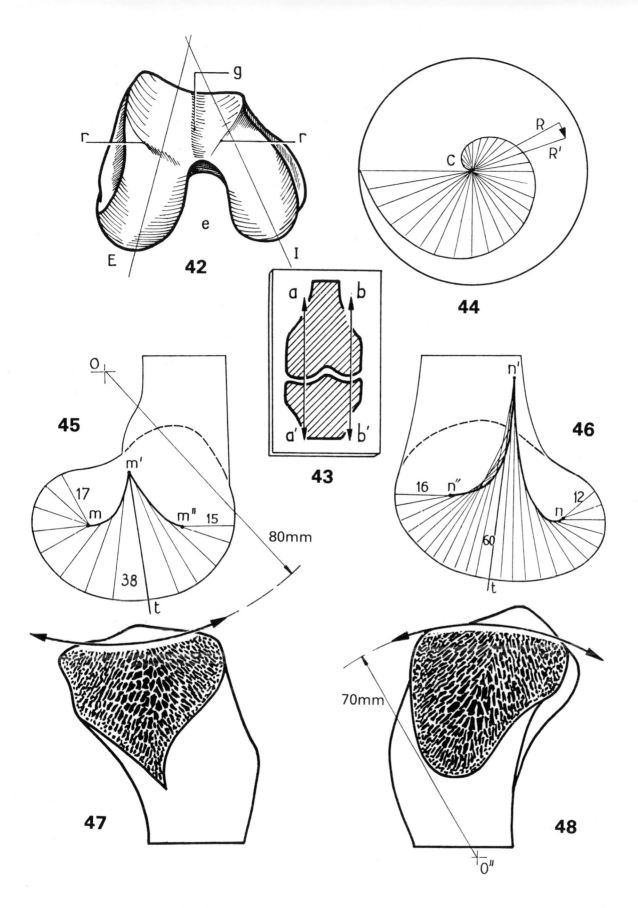

42

43

44

45

46

47

48

FACTORS DETERMINING THE SHAPE OF THE DISTAL FEMUR

With the use of a **mechanical model** (fig. 49) I showed in 1967 that the outlines of the femoral trochlea and condyles are **geometrical entities** determined, on the one hand, by the interaction between the cruciate ligaments and their femoral and tibial attachments and, on the other, by the relationships among the ligamentum patellae, the patella and patellar retinacula. When this model is set in motion (fig. 50), the profiles of the femoral condyles and trochlea are outlined by the *envelope of the successive positions of the tibial condyles and of the patella* (fig. 51).

The **posterior part of the condylo-trochlear profile**, related to the tibia (fig. 51), is moulded by the successive positions (1 to 5) of the tibial plateau, 'slavishly' bound to the femur by the medial (short dashes) and the lateral (long dashes) cruciate ligaments. Each ligament sweeps an arc of a circle with its centre located at the femoral insertion and radius equal to the length of the ligament. Thus, in extreme flexion, the joint space gapes anteriorly owing to relaxation of the medial cruciate at the end of flexion, while the lateral cruciate is stretched.

The **anterior part of the condylo-trochlear profile**, related to the patella, (fig. 52), is moulded by the successive positions (1 to 6) of the patella bound to the femur by the retinacula and to the tibia by the **ligamentum patellae**.

Between the anterior (patellar) and the posterior (tibial) parts of the condylotrochlear profile there is a *transition point t* (figs. 45 and 46), representing the boundary between the femoropatellar and the femorotibial joints.

By changing the geometrical relationships of the cruciate system it is possible to trace a *family of curves* for the condyles and the trochlea, and this underlies the uniqueness of each knee. Geometrically speaking, no two knees are alike; hence the difficulty of producing a perfect prosthesis for a particular knee. Prostheses can only be more or less faithful approximations.

The same problems arise when the cruciates are subjected to plastic operations or prosthetic replacements. For example (fig. 53), if the tibial insertion of the medial cruciate is displaced anteriorly, the circle described by its femoral insertion will also be displaced anteriorly (fig. 54), giving rise to a **new condylar profile** lying within the original. This causes some degree of **mechanical 'play'** in the joint with undue erosion of the cartilaginous surfaces.

A. Menschik of Vienna has confirmed these ideas by a purely geometrical analysis.

Obviously, this theory of geometrical determination of the condylotrochlear profile is based on the **isometry hypothesis**, i.e. the constancy of length of cruciate ligaments, which is not quite true. Nonetheless, it explains many facts and acts as a guide in the development of new operations on these ligaments.

More recently, Frain et al, using a **mathematical model** based on an anatomical study of 20 knees, have confirmed the idea of the curve-envelope and of the multiplicity of the centres of instantaneous movements and have stressed the functional relationship between the cruciate and the collateral ligaments. The computer tracing of the velocity vectors at each point of contact between femur and tibia reproduces exactly the envelope generating the condylar profile.

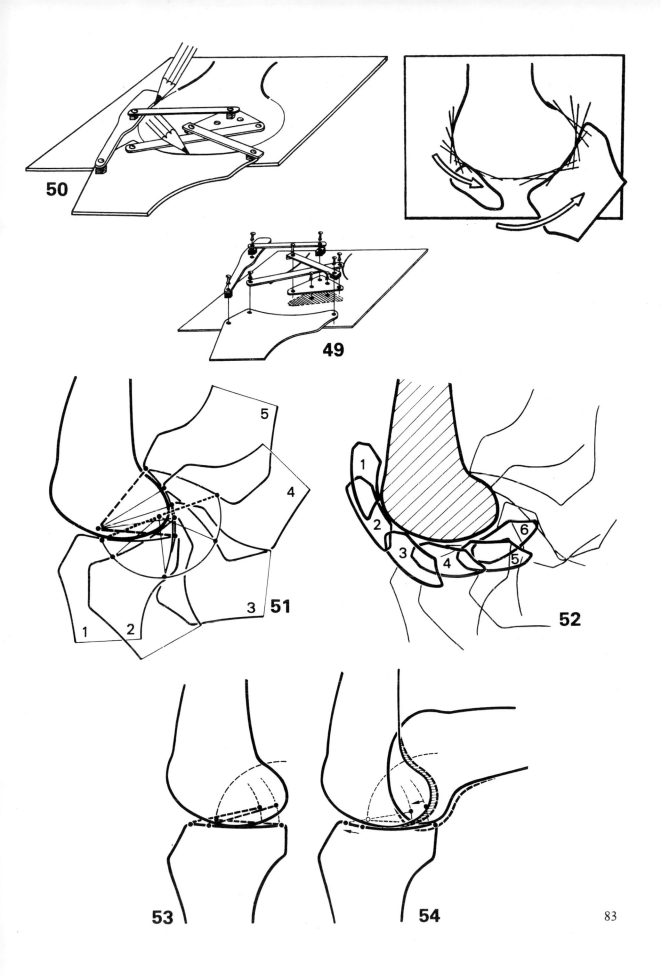

50

49

51

52

53

54

83

MOVEMENTS OF THE FEMORAL CONDYLES ON THE TIBIAL PLATEAU DURING FLEXION AND EXTENSION

The rounded shape of the condyles could suggest that they roll over the tibial condyles, but this is wrong. In fact when **a wheel rolls on the ground without sliding** (fig. 55), *to each point on the ground corresponds a single point on the wheel* so that the distance covered on the ground (OO") is exactly equal to the portion of the circumference which has rolled over the ground (distance between the point marked by a triangle and that marked by a rectangle). If this were so (fig. 56), after a certain measure of flexion (position II) the femoral condyle would tip over behind the tibial condyle—i.e. dislocation of the joint—or else the tibial condyle would need to be longer. The possibility of a simple rolling movement of the femoral condyle is precluded by the fact that *the length of the circumference of the femoral condyle is twice as great as the length of the tibial condyle.*

Let us now assume that **the wheel slides without rolling** (fig. 57): *therefore to one point on the ground corresponds a segment of the circumference of the wheel.* This is what happens when a car wheel 'spins' when starting on a frosty road. Such a type of sliding movement could conceivably explain the movements of the femoral condyle on the tibial condyle (fig. 58). So to one point on the tibial condyle would correspond all the points of the condylar surface. But it is clear that under these conditions *flexion would be prematurely checked by* the impact of the femur on the posterior border of the tibial condyle (arrow).

It is also possible to imagine that **the wheel rolls and slides simultaneously** (fig. 59): it skids but still moves forward. Therefore to the distance covered on the ground (OO') corresponds a length much greater on the surface of the wheel (between the black diamond and the black triangle) than could be obtained by 'unrolling' the wheel on the ground (between black diamond and white triangle).

The experiment performed by the Weber brothers (fig. 60) in 1836 showed that the last mechanism actually operated in life. For various positions between extreme extension and extreme flexion they marked on the cartilage the corresponding points of contact between the femoral and tibial condyles. They then noted on the one hand that *the point of contact on the tibia moved backwards during flexion* (black triangle: extension, black diamond: flexion) and on the other hand that the distance between the points of contact marked on the femoral condyle was twice as long as that between the corresponding points on the tibial condyle. This experiment proves indisputably that the **femoral condyle rolls and slides simultaneously over the tibial condyle.** This is after all the only way that posterior dislocation of the femoral condyle can be avoided while a greater range of flexion remains possible (160°: compare flexion in figs. 58 and 60).

More recent experiments (Strasser 1917) have shown that the ratio of rolling to sliding varies during flexion and extension. Starting from full extension *the femoral condyle begins to roll without sliding and then the sliding movement becomes progressively more important so that at the end of flexion the condyle slides without rolling.*

Finally, the length over which pure rolling takes place **varies with the femoral condyle:**
for the medial condyle (fig. 61) pure rolling occurs only during the first 10° to 15° of flexion;
for the lateral condyle (fig. 62) this rolling goes on until 20° flexion is reached.

Therefore the lateral condyle rolls far more than the medial and this partly explains why the distance covered by the lateral femoral condyle over the corresponding tibial condyle is greater than that covered by the medial condyle. This important fact will be considered again in relation to automatic rotation (p. 144).

It is also interesting to note that the 15° to 20° of initial rolling corresponds to the normal range of the movements of flexion and extension during ordinary walking.

Frain et al have shown that to every point along the path traced by the femoral condyles there correspond, on the one hand, the centre of the **osculatory circle** representing the *centre of curvature of the condyle* at this point and, on the other, the *centre of the path of motion*, representing the point around which the femur rotates with respect to the tibia. It is only when these two centres coincide that a pure rolling movement occurs. The degree of sliding relative to rolling varies directly with the distance between these two centres.

84

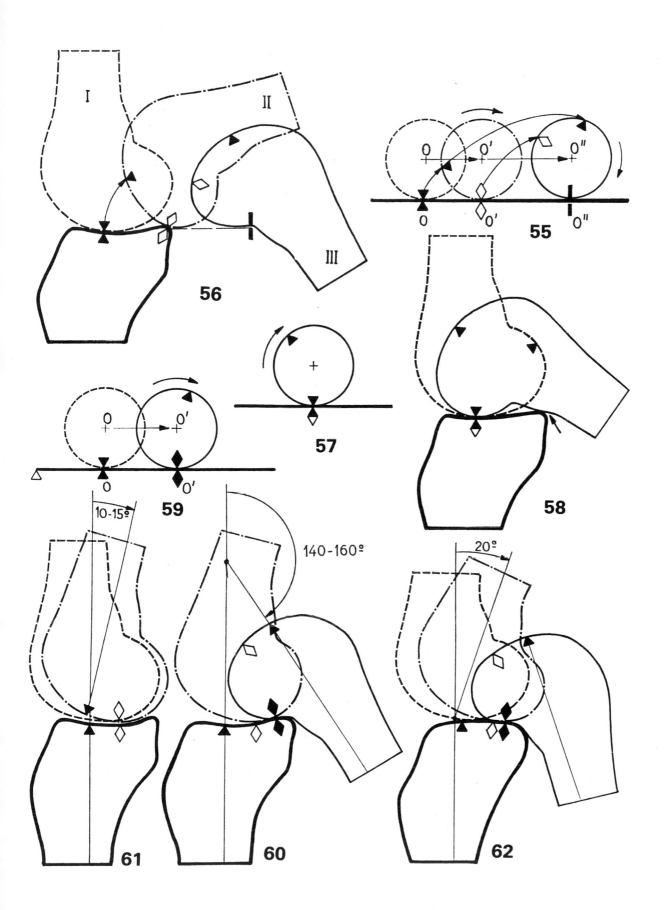

55

56

57

58

59

10-15°

140-160°

20°

61

60

62

MOVEMENTS OF THE FEMORAL CONDYLES ON THE TIBIAL PLATEAU DURING AXIAL ROTATION

It will become apparent later why axial rotation can only take place when the knee is flexed. **In the neutral position for axial rotation** (fig. 63), with the knee flexed, the posterior part of the femoral condyles is in contact with *the middle part of the tibial condyles*. This is clearly illustrated by the diagram (fig. 64), where the outline of the femoral condyles (transparent) can be seen superimposed on the outline of the tibia condyles (striped). It is also clear from this diagram that with flexion of the knee the intercondylar tibial tubercles have moved clear of the intercondylar notch of the femur, where they normally lodge during extension (this is one of the reasons preventing axial rotation during extension).

During **lateral rotation** of the tibia on the femur (fig. 65) the lateral femoral condyle moves forward over the lateral tibial condyle while the medial femoral condyle moves backward over the medial tibial condyle (fig. 66).

During **medial rotation** (fig. 67) the converse takes place: the lateral femoral condyle moves posteriorly and the medial femoral condyle moves anteriorly over their respective tibial condyles (fig. 68).

The **anteroposterior movements of the femoral condyles** over their respective tibial condyles vary with the condyle:

the **medial femoral condyle** (fig. 69) moves relatively little (1);

the **lateral femoral condyle** (fig. 70), on the other hand, moves nearly twice as much (L) on the convex lateral tibial condyle. As it moves anteroposteriorly it 'climbs' the anterior slope of the convex tibial condyle to reach the 'top of the mountain' and then goes down the posterior slope. Thus the femoral condyle changes its 'altitude' (e).

The difference in the shape of the two tibial condyles is reflected in **the configuration of the inter-condylar spines**. A horizontal section of these spines at level XX' (fig. 71) shows that the lateral aspect of the lateral spine is *convex* anteroposteriorly (like the lateral tibial condyle) whereas the medial surface of the medial spine is *concave* (like the medial tibial condyle): the medial spine is also *clearly higher than the lateral spine*. As a result of these two features, the medial spine juts out as a stop-shoulder against which the medial femoral condyle knocks, while the lateral condyle easily moves past the corresponding spine. Therefore **the real axis of axial rotation** does not pass between the two spines but *through the medial spine* which constitutes the central pivot of the joint. This displacement of the 'centre' medially is reflected in the greater movement of the lateral condyle as shown previously.

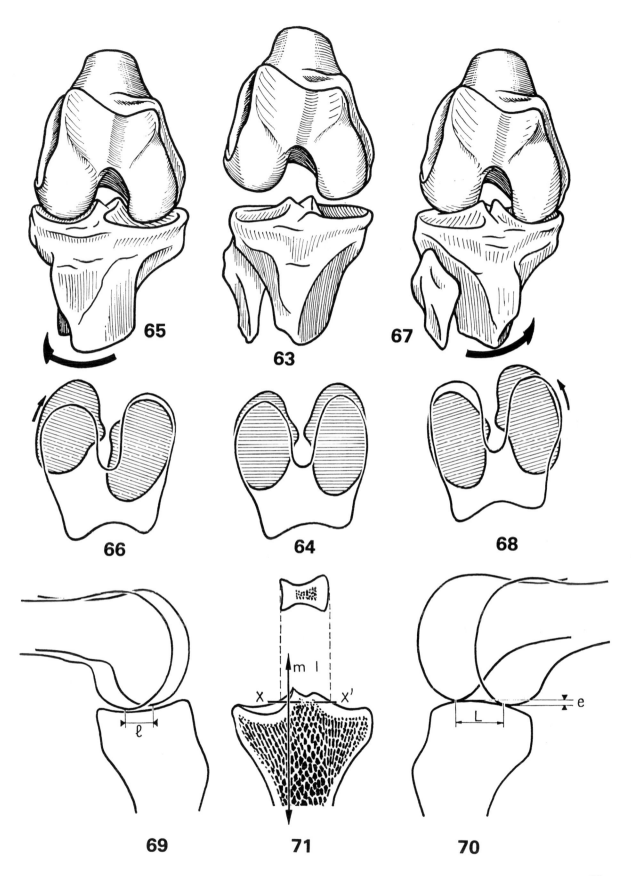

65

63

67

66

64

68

69

71

70

THE CAPSULE OF THE KNEE

The articular capsule is a fibrous sleeve, which invests the distal end of the femur and the proximal end of the tibia, keeps the two bones in contact and forms the non-bony wall of the articular space. Its deep surface is covered by **synovium**.

The general form of the capsule (fig. 72) can be easily understood if it is compared to a *cylinder* which is invaginated posteriorly (as shown by the white arrow). This leads to the formation of a *partition* in the sagittal plane, which almost divides the cavity into a medial and a lateral half; its relations to the cruciate ligaments will be studied later (p. 116). On the anterior surface of the cylinder a *window* is cut to receive the patella. The upper and lower ends of the cylinder are attached to the femur and the tibia respectively.

The **attachment of the capsule to the tibia** is relatively simple (fig. 73). It is inserted (dotted line) into the anterior, lateral and medial borders of the articular surface. Posteromedially it blends into the tibial insertion of the posterior cruciate ligament; posterolaterally it lines the edge of the lateral condyle posterior to the tibial spine and joins the tibial insertion of the posterior cruciate ligament. The capsule does not extend between the cruciate ligaments and the gap is filled by synovium lining the cruciate ligaments, which can thus be viewed as thickenings of the articular capsule in the intercondylar fossa.

The femoral attachment of the capsule is slightly more complex (figs. 74 to 77):

anteriorly (fig. 74), the capsule is attached to the bone along the edges of the shallow fossa overlying the patellar surface (7). At this point the capsule forms a deep recess (figs. 76 to 77), known as the *suprapatellar bursa* (5); its importance will emerge later (p. 98);

medially and laterally (figs. 74 to 75) it is inserted along the margins of the patellar surface forming the *parapatellar recesses* (p. 98) and then along the edges of the articular surfaces of the condyles like a *banister* (8); on the lateral condyle the capsular insertion lies above the insertion of the popliteus tendon (P), which is therefore *intracapsular* (see figs, 147 and 232);

posteriorly and superiorly (fig. 75) the capsule is inserted round the posterosuperior border of the articular surfaces of the condyles, just distal to the origins of the two heads of the gastrocnemius (g). The capsule therefore lines the deep surface of these muscles and separates them from the condyles; in this area the capsule is thickened to form what can be called 'condylar plates' (6) (p. 110);

in the intercondylar notch (figs. 76 to 77: the femur has been cut in the sagittal plane) the capsule is attached to the opposing surfaces of the condyles along the articular cartilage and then to the depths of the notch, which it bridges. Its insertion in to the medial condyle (fig. 76) runs *below the femoral attachment of the posterior cruciate ligament* (4). Its insertion in to the lateral condyle (3) lies *between the articular cartilage and the femoral attachment of the anterior cruciate ligament* (fig. 77).

Here too the insertion of the cruciate ligaments blends into that of the capsule, reinforcing the latter.

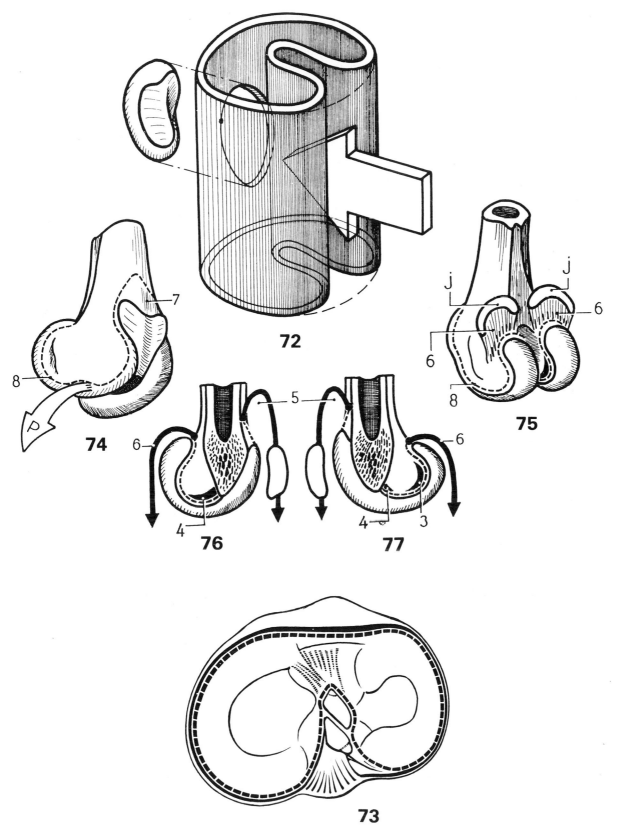

72

74

75

76

77

73

THE INFRAPATELLAR FOLD, THE PLICAE AND THE CAPACITY OF THE JOINT

The empty space, bounded by the anterior intercondylar fossa of the tibia, the ligamentum patellae and the inferior aspect of the patellar surface of the femur, is filled by a considerable pad of adipose tissue known as **the infrapatellar pad** (fig. 78). This pad (1) has the shape of a *quadrangular pyramid* with its base resting on the posterior surface (2) of the ligamentum patellae (3) and overlapping the anterior part of the anterior intercondylar fossa. Its superior aspect (4) is strengthened by a fibro-adipose band attached to the apex of the patella and lying in the intercondylar notch (fig. 78 and 79): this band is *the infrapatellar fold* (5). At the sides (fig. 79: the knee has been opened anteriorly and the patella tilted) the infrapatellar pad extends superiorly along the inferior part of the sides of the patella in the form of two fringe-like folds of fibro-adipose tissue, i.e. *the alar folds* (6). The infrapatellar pad acts as a 'stopgap' in the anterior compartment of the joint. During flexion it is compressed by the ligamentum patellae and spreads out on either side of the patellar apex.

The infrapatellar pad is the vestige of the *median septum*, which divides the joint into two cavities in the embryo up to four months. In the adult, there is normally a gap (fig. 78) between the infrapatellar pad and the median septum formed by the capsule (arrow I). Therefore the lateral and medial halves of the joint cavity communicate with each other via this gap as well as via the space lying above the pad (arrow II) and deep to the patella. Occasionally the median septum persists in the adult and these only communicate above the infrapatellar pad. This structure is also known as the *infrapatellar plica* or *ligamentum muscosum*.

The synovium of the knee joint includes (fig. 83) **three plicae** (recesses), which are variable but quite common (seen in 85 per cent of cases, according to Dupont). These plicae, now well recognized owing to **arthroscopy**, consist of:

the **infrapatellar plica** (5), extending beyond the infrapatellar pad, is present in 65·5 per cent of cases.

the **suprapatellar plica** (6), seen in 55·5 per cent of cases, forms a horizontal partition superior to the patella. It can be partial or complete, in the latter case isolating the suprapatellar bursa from the joint cavity. Under these conditions it can give rise to hydrarthrosis ('water on the knee').

the **mediopatellar plica** (7), seen in 24 per cent of cases, forms an incomplete shelf between femur and patella. It can cause pain when its free border rubs against the medial border of the medial condyle. Arthroscopic resection is curative.

The **capacity of the joint cavity** varies under normal and pathological conditions. An effusion—hydrarthrosis or haemarthrosis—increases this capacity substantially (fig. 80), provided it accumulates *gradually*; the fluid collects in the suprapatellar bursa (SP), in the parapatellar recesses and posteriorly in the gastrocnemius bursa (GB) deep to the 'condylar plates'.

The distribution of the fluid within the cavity varies according to the position of the knee. **In extension** (fig. 81) the gastrocnemius bursa is compressed by tension of the gastrocnemius and the fluid *moves anteriorly* where it collects into the suprapatellar bursa and the parapatellar recesses. **In flexion** (fig. 82) these become compressed by tension of the quadriceps and the fluid *moves posteriorly*. Between full flexion and full extension there *is a position of so-called maximal capacity* (fig. 80), where the fluid within the cavity is under least tension. This position of semi-flexion is assumed by patients with an effusion as it is the least painful.

Normally the amount of *synovial fluid* is *very small* amounting to a few cubic centimetres. However, the movements of flexion and extension ensure that the articular surfaces are constantly bathed by fresh synovial fluid and thus assist in the proper nutrition of the cartilage and especially in the lubrication of the surfaces in contact.

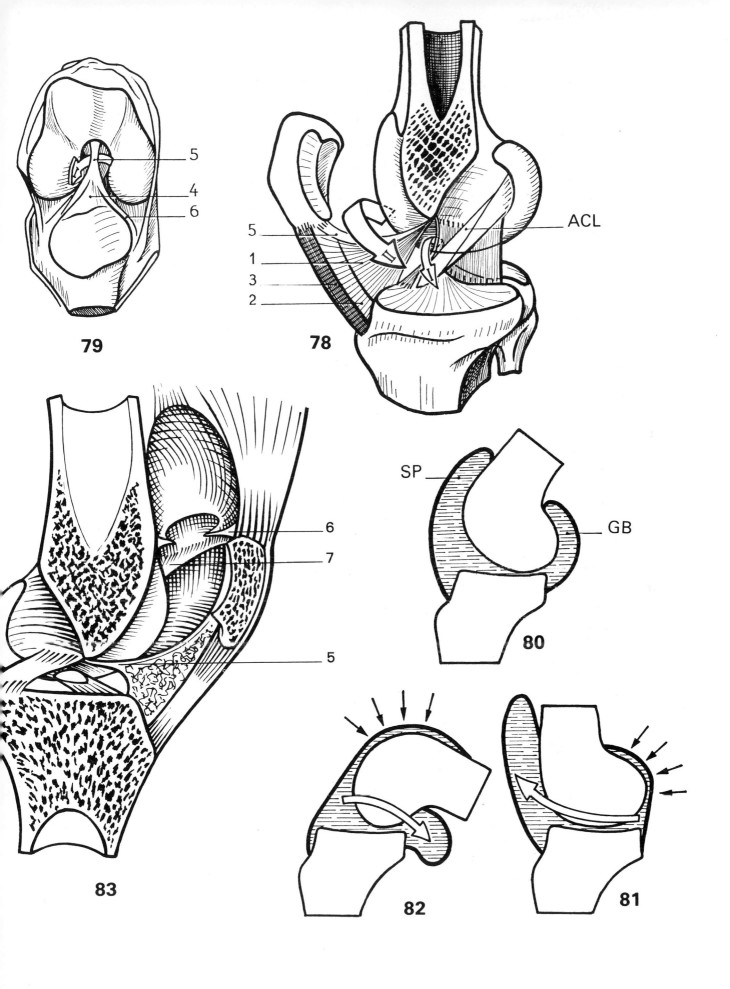

79

78

5
1
3
2

5
4
6

ACL

83

6
7

5

SP

GB

80

82

81

THE MENISCI OF THE KNEE

The lack of congruence of the articular surfaces (p. 80) is corrected by the interposition of **the menisci or semilunar cartilages,** the shape of which can easily be understood (fig. 84). If a sphere (S) is placed on a plane (P) contact occurs only tangentially with respect to the sphere. To increase the area of contact between the sphere and the plane, it will suffice to place between them a ring equal in volume to that bounded by the sphere, the plane P and the cylinder C which lies tangential to the sphere. Such a ring (shaded) has precisely the shape of a meniscus, *triangular in cross-section*, with the following **three surfaces** (fig. 85: the menisci have been lifted off the tibial condyles):

the superior surface (1), concave, in contact with the femoral condyles;

the peripheral surface (2), cylindrical in shape, adherent to the deep surface of the capsule (shown by the vertical stripes);

the inferior surface (3), almost plane, resting on the edges of the medial (MTC) and the lateral (LTC) tibial condyles.

These rings are incomplete in the region of the intercondylar tubercles of the tibia so that they are *crescent-shaped* with an anterior and a posterior horn. The horns of the lateral meniscus come closer to each other so that *the meniscus is almost a complete circle* (in the shape of an O) whereas the medial meniscus is *a half-moon*, i.e. C-shaped.

These menisci are not unattached between the femoral and tibial surfaces and *have important attachments from the functional point of view*:

the deep surface of the *capsule* (fig. 86), as seen previously, is attached to the menisci;

each horn is anchored to the *tibial condyle* in the anterior and posterior intercondylar fossae respectively:

the anterior horn of the lateral meniscus (4) just in front of the lateral intercondylar tubercle; the posterior horn of the lateral meniscus (5) just behind the lateral intercondylar tubercle; the posterior horn of the medial meniscus (7) in the posteromedial angle of the posterior intercondylar fossa; the medial horn of the medial meniscus (6) in the anteromedial angle of the anterior intercondylar fossa;

the two anterior horns are linked by the *transverse ligament of the knee* (8), which is itself attached to the patella by strands of the infrapatellar pad;

fibrous bands run from the lateral edges of the patella (P) to the lateral borders of each meniscus forming the *menisco-patellar fibres* (9);

the *medial collateral ligament* (MCL) of the knee is attached by its deep fibres to the internal border of the medial meniscus;

the *lateral collateral ligament* (LCL), however, is separated from its corresponding meniscus by the tendon of the popliteus (Pop) which sends a fibrous expansion (10) to the posterior border of the *lateral meniscus* (LM);

the *semimembranosus tendon* (11) also sends a fibrous expansion to the posterior edge of the *medial meniscus* (MM);

finally separate fibres of the posterior cruciate ligament are inserted into the posterior horn of the lateral meniscus forming the *menisco-femoral ligament* (12). There are also a few fibres of the anterior cruciate ligament inserted into the *anterior horn of the medial meniscus* (fig. 152).

The coronal section (fig. 86) and the medial (fig. 87) and lateral (fig. 88) parasagittal sections show how the menisci are placed *between the tibial and femoral condyles*, except at the centre of each tibial condyle and in the region of the intercondylar tubercles, and also how the menisci divide the joint into two compartments: the suprameniscal and the inframeniscal compartments (fig. 86).

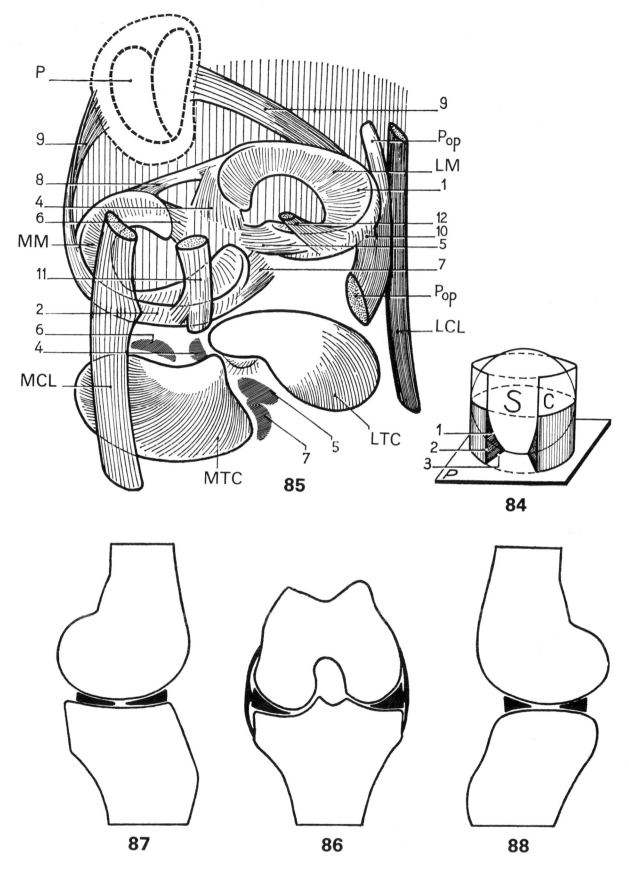

85

P

9

8

4

6

MM

11

2

6

4

MCL

MTC

9

P_op

LM

1

12

10

5

7

P_op

LCL

LTC

5

7

84

S C

1

2

3

P

87

86

88

MOVEMENTS OF THE MENISCI DURING FLEXION AND EXTENSION

As shown before (p. 82), the point of contact between the femoral and tibial condyles moves posteriorly during flexion and anteriorly during extension; the menisci follow these movements, as is easily demonstrated in an anatomical preparation containing only the ligaments and the menisci. *In extension* (fig. 89), the *posterior part of the tibial condyle becomes exposed*, especially the lateral condyle (LTC). *In flexion* (fig. 90) *the menisci (medial and lateral) come to overlie the posterior part of the tibial condyles*, especially the lateral meniscus which reaches as far as the posterior border of the lateral condyle.

When the menisci are viewed from above it is obvious that starting from the position of extension (fig. 91), *the menisci move posteriorly unequally*; in flexion (fig. 92), the lateral meniscus (LM) has receded twice as far as the medial meniscus (MM). In fact, the posterior displacement of the medial meniscus is 6 mm., that of the lateral meniscus 12 mm.

It is also clear from these diagrams that, while they recede, *the menisci become distorted*. This is due to the fact that they have two fixed points, their anterior and posterior horns, while the rest of the structure is freely mobile. The lateral meniscus undergoes a greater degree of distortion and posterior displacement because its horns are attached much closer together.

The menisci play an important part as *an elastic coupling which transmits any compression forces* between the femur and the tibia (black arrows, figs. 94 and 95). It is worth nothing that during extension the femoral condyles present their *greatest radii of curvature* to the tibial condyles (fig. 93) and the menisci are *tightly interposed* between the articular surfaces. These two factors *promote the transmission of compression forces* during full knee extension. On the other hand, during flexion, the femoral condyles display their shortest radii of curvature (fig. 96) and the menisci are only partially in contact with these condyles (fig. 98). These two factors, along with relaxation of the collateral ligaments (p. 104), *favour mobility at the expense of stability*.

After defining the movements of the menisci, the factors involved in these movements call for discussion. These factors fall into *two groups*: passive and active.

There is only **one passive element** involved in the displacement of the menisci: the *femoral condyles push the menisci anteriorly* just as a cherrystone is pushed forward between two fingers. This apparently over-simple mechanism is perfectly obvious when one studies an anatomical preparation where all the connections of the menisci have been severed except for the attachments of their horns (figs. 89 and 90). The surfaces are slippery and the 'wedge' of the meniscus is pushed anteriorly between the 'wheel' of the femoral condyle and the 'ground' of the tibial condyle (as a lock mechanism it is wholly inefficient).

The **active mechanisms** are numerous:

during extension (figs. 94 and 95), the menisci are pulled forward by the *meniscopatellar fibres* (1), which are stretched by the anterior movement of the patella (p. 102) and this draws the transverse ligament forward. In addition, the posterior horn of the lateral meniscus is pulled anteriorly (fig. 95) by the tension developed in the *meniscofemoral ligament* (2), as the posterior cruciate ligament becomes taut (p. 124);

during flexion, the medial meniscus (fig. 97) is drawn posteriorly by *the semimembranosus expansion* which is attached to its posterior edge, while the anterior horn is pulled anteriorly by the *fibres of the anterior cruciate ligament* attached to it (4); the *lateral meniscus* (fig. 98) is drawn posteriorly by the popliteus expansion (5).

The critical role played by the menisci in the transmission of compressive forces between femur and tibia was underestimated until it was noted that the first patients subjected to 'prophylactic' meniscectomy were developing premature osteoarthritis. Considerable progress has followed the advent of **arthroscopy**. First, it allowed better evaluation of doubtful meniscal lesions identified arthrographically (the false-positives) and put an end to 'wildcat' meniscectomies (some menisci were removed to find out if they were abnormal!) Second, it led to tailored meniscectomies with removal of damaged segments causing mechanical embarrassment or injury to the articular cartilage. Third, it brought home the lesson that *detection of the meniscal lesion is only part of the diagnosis*, since often it is ligamentous failure that underlies both the meniscal and the cartilaginous lesion.

94

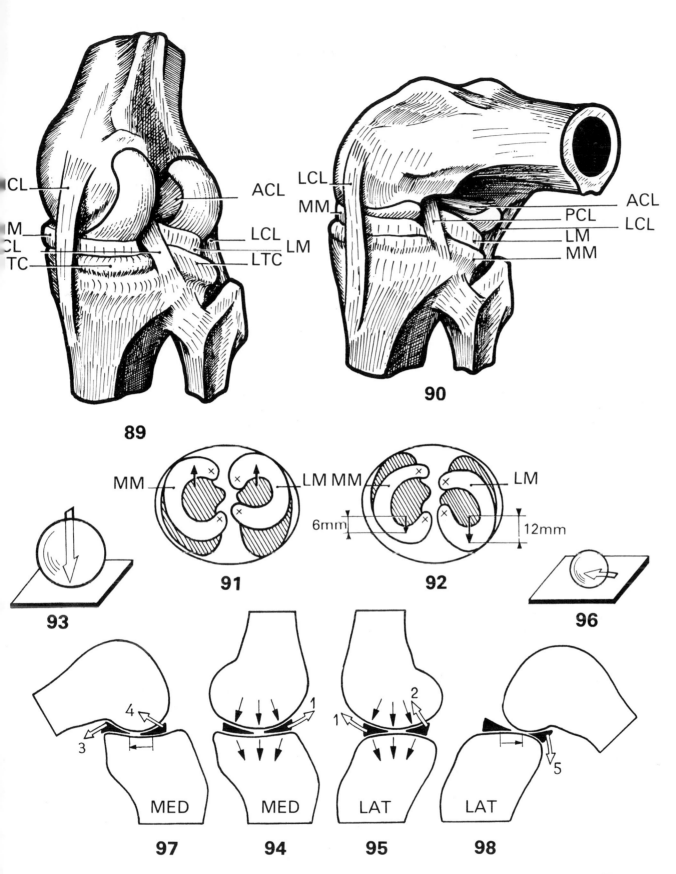

CL

M
CL
TC

ACL

LCL
LM
LTC

89

LCL
MM

ACL
PCL
LCL
LM
MM

90

MM

LM MM

LM

6mm

12mm

91

92

93

96

4
3

1

2
1

5

MED

MED

LAT

LAT

97

94

95

98

MOVEMENTS OF THE MENISCI DURING AXIAL ROTATION; LESIONS OF THE MENISCI

During the movements of axial rotation, the menisci follow *exactly* the displacements of femoral condyles (p. 86). Starting from the neutral position (fig. 99) they can be seen to move on the tibial condyles in the opposite direction.:

during lateral rotation (fig. 100), the lateral meniscus (LM) is pulled towards the anterior part (1) of the tibial condyle while the medial meniscus (MM) is drawn posteriorly (2);

during medial rotation (fig. 101), the medial meniscus (MM) moves forward (3) while the lateral meniscus (LM) recedes (4).

Here again the menisci during their movements *become distorted* about their fixed points, i.e. the attachments of their horns. The total range of the movement of the lateral meniscus (1+4) is twice as great as that of the medial meniscus (2+3).

These displacements of the menisci during axial rotation are mostly passive—being drawn by the femoral condyles—but there is also an active mechanism involved. The *meniscopatellar fibres become taut* as a result of movement of the patella in relation to the tibia (p. 102) and this tension in these fibres draws one of the menisci anteriorly.

During movements of the knee **the menisci can be injured** if they fail to follow the movements of the femoral condyles on the tibial condyles; they are thus 'caught unawares' in an abnormal position and are 'squashed between the anvil and the hammer'. This happens, for instance, **during violent extension of the knee** (i.e. kicking a football): one of the menisci fails to move forwards (fig. 102) and is caught between the femoral and tibial condyles as the tibia is forcefully applied to the femur. This mechanism, very common among footballers, leads to *transverse tears* (fig. 107) or to *detachment of the anterior horn* (b), which then becomes folded on itself. The other mechanism producing lesions of the menisci involves a **twisting movement of the knee joint** (fig. 103), which combines *lateral displacement* (1) and *lateral rotation* (2). The medial meniscus is then pulled towards the centre of the joint under the convexity of the medial femoral condyle; when the joint is extended it is caught off guard and crushed between the two condyles with the following possible consequences: (a) a *longitudinal splitting of the meniscus* (fig. 104) or (b) a *complete detachment of the meniscus from the capsule* (fig. 105) or (c) a *complex tear of the meniscus* (fig. 106). In all these longitudinal lesions the central free part of the meniscus can rear itself up into the intercondylar notch so that the meniscus assumes the shape of a *bucket-handle*. This type of lesion is very common among footballers (during falls on a flexed leg) and among miners who have to work crouched in narrow seams of coal.

Another cause of meniscal injury is rupture of a cruciate ligament, e.g. the anterior cruciate (fig. 108). The medial femoral condyle is no longer held back posteriorly and 'clips' the posterior horn of the medial meniscus, which is pulled off its capsular attachment posteriorly or gets torn horizontally (inset).

As soon as a meniscus is torn, the injured part fails to follow the normal movements and becomes wedged between the femoral and tibial condyles. The knee as a result *'locks'* in a position of flexion, which is more marked the more posterior the rupture; *full extension is then impossible.*

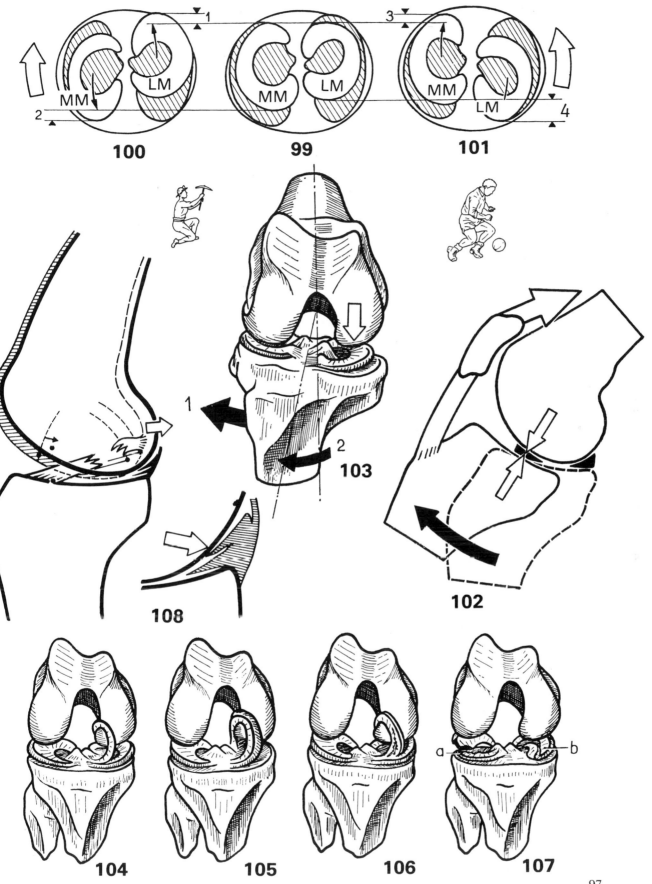

100 **99** **101**

103

108

102

104 **105** **106** **107**

97

MOVEMENTS OF THE PATELLA ON THE FEMUR

The extensor apparatus of the knee slides on the lower end of the femur like **a cable on a pulley** (fig. 109a). The patellar surface of the femur and the intercondylar notch (fig. 110) effectively form a deep vertical gutter (fig. 109b), in the depths of which slides the patella. Thus the force of the quadriceps, directed obliquely superiorly and *slightly laterally*, is turned into a *strictly vertical force*.

The normal movement of the patella on the femur during flexion is therefore a vertical displacement along the central groove of the femoral patellar surface down to the intercondylar notch (fig. 111: based on X-ray studies). Thus the patella moves downwards *over a distance equal to twice its length* (8 cm.), while turning on itself about a transverse axis. Its deep surface, which looks directly posteriorly in extension (A), faces superiorly when the patella, at the end of its downward displacement in full flexion (B), comes to lie against the femoral condyles. This movement can thus be called '**circumferential displacement**'.

This important displacement is only possible when the patella is attached to the femur by connections of sufficient length. The capsule forms three recesses in relation to the patella (fig. 111) superiorly, the *suprapatellar bursa* (SP) and on either side the *parapatellar recesses* (PRP). When the patella slides under the condyles from A to B these three recesses become unpleated and the distance XX' can become XX'' (i.e. four times greater) only because of the length of the suprapatellar bursa. Likewise, the distance YY' can become YY'' (i.e. twice as great) because of the length of the parapatellar recesses.

When inflammatory adhesions develop in these recesses their cavities are obliterated and *the patella is tightly held against the femur* (i.e. XX' and YY' became inextensible) and cannot slide down the central groove. This is one of the causes of the post-traumatic or post-infective '*stiff knee*'.

During its downward displacement the patella is followed by the *infrapatellar pad* (fig. 112) which moves from position ZZ' to position ZZ'', i.e. through an angle of 180°. When the patella is displaced superiorly during extension, the suprapatellar bursa would be caught between patella and femur, were it not drawn upwards by the *articularis genu muscle* (AGM) (tensor of the suprapatellar bursa), whic arises from the deep surface of the vastus intermedius.

Normally the patella moves only in the vertical plane and not transversely. It is in fact very strongly applied to its groove (fig. 113) by the quadriceps, the more so as the degree of flexion increases (a). At the end of extension (b) this appositional force is diminished and in hyperextension (c) it even tends to be reversed, i.e. to separate the patella from the femur. At this point (d) the patella tends *to be driven laterally* because the quadriceps tendon and the ligamentum patellae form *an angle obtuse laterally*. Lateral dislocation of the patella is prevented by the lateral lip of the patellar surface of the femur (fig. 114) *which is distinctly more prominent than the medial lip* (difference=e). If, as a result of a congenital malformation (fig. 115), this lateral lip is underdeveloped (i.e. is as prominent as the medial lip or less prominent) the patella is no longer held in and dislocates laterally during full extension. This is the mechanism underlying *recurrent dislocation of the patella*.

Both lateral rotation of the tibia under the femur and genu valgum close the angle between the quadriceps tendon and the ligamentum patellae and increase the lateral vector of force promoting lateral instability of the patella. These conditions thus set the stage for lateral dislocations and subluxations, chondromalacia patellae and lateral femoro-patellar osteoarthritis.

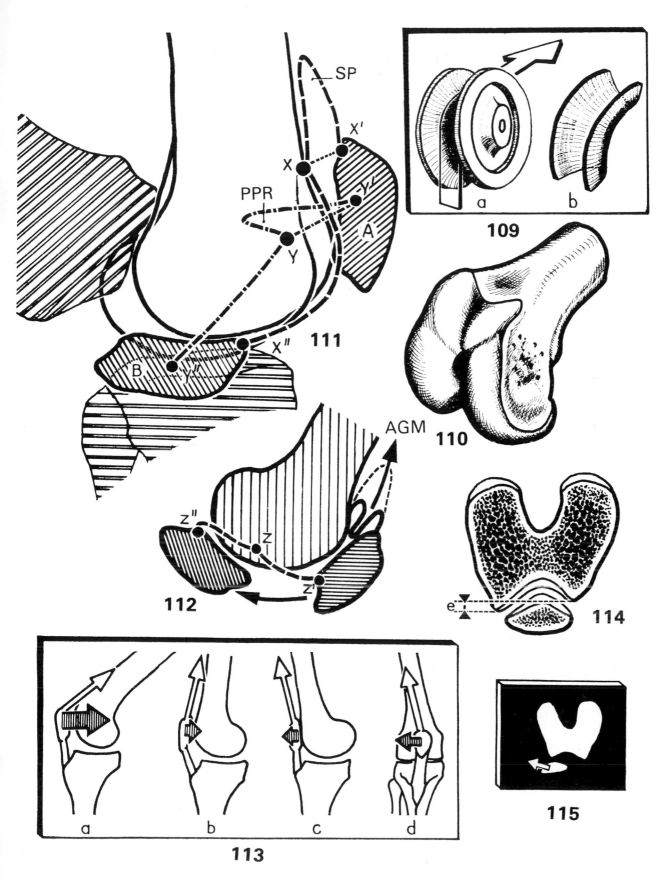

109

111

110

112

AGM

114

113

115

99

FEMORO-PATELLAR RELATIONSHIPS

The posterior aspect of the patella (fig. 116), particularly the median vertical ridge, is coated with thick cartilage (4–5 mm. thick), which is **the thickest in the body**. This is due to the tremendous pressures (300 kg. and even more during weightlifting) applied to the patella, when the quadriceps contracts with the knee flexed, as when one goes down stairs or rises from the squatting position.

On either side of the median ridge there are two biconcave facets:

the **lateral**, related to the lateral aspect of the trochlea;

the **medial**, related to the medial aspect. It is further subdivided by a low oblique ridge into a **main facet** and an **accessory facet**, which lies at the superomedial angle and is related to the medial edge of the intercondylar fossa during extreme flexion.

As the patella moves **vertically** along the trochlea during flexion (fig. 117), it comes into contact with the trochlea on its inferior aspect in full extension, on its central aspect at 30° flexion and on its superior and superomedial aspects in full flexion. It is thus possible to determine the **critical angle of flexion** from the topography of the cartilaginous lesions and, conversely, to predict the site of the lesions by determining the **angle at which flexion becomes painful**.

Up to now, the femoropatellar joint was studied with the use of axial radiographs of the patella or by successive films of the joint space (fig. 118). Each film shows **both patellae** with the knee flexed at 30° (A), 60° (B) and 90° (C) to allow complete visualization of the joint.

From these films of the joint space the following observations can be made:

the *central location of the patella*, especially on the film taken with the knee flexed at 30°, is assessed by the interlocking of the patellar ridge and the trochlear groove and the overhanging of the lateral border of the trochlea by the lateral edge of the patella. By comparison, a diagnosis of lateral subluxation can be made.

thinning of the joint space, especially laterally, can be evaluated using calipers and by comparison with the other normal knee. Cartilage erosion can thus be detected in advanced osteoarthritis.

subchondral osteosclerosis of the lateral facet, indicating the presence of *abnormal lateral stresses* on the joint.

lateral displacement of the anterior tibial tubercle with respect to the trochlear groove, seen only in radiographs taken with the knee flexed at 30° (A) or 60° (B), indicates **lateral rotation** of the tibia on the femur caused by subluxation and abnormal lateral stresses on the joint.

Nowadays, with **computed tomography** the femoropatellar joint can be studied in **full extension** or even in hyperextension, which was impossible to do radiologically. These scans demonstrate lateral subluxation of the patella in positions where the force of articular coaptation is nil or even negative and thus allows the detection of *minor degrees of joint instability*.

With **arthroscopy** dynamic imbalances in the joint can be recognized as well as cartilaginous lesions undetectable on axial radiographs.

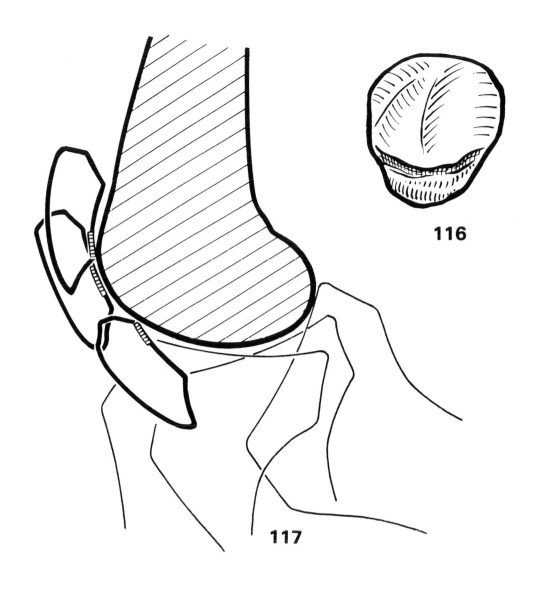

116

117

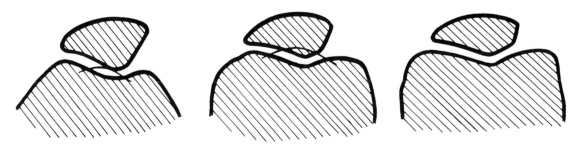

118

101

MOVEMENTS OF THE PATELLA ON THE TIBIA

One could imagine the patella welded to the tibia in the form of an olecranon process as at the elbow (fig. 119). This arrangement would prevent all movements of the patella relative to the tibia and would notably curtail its mobility and even prevent any axial rotation.

The patella in fact exhibits **two types of movement** relative to the tibia, one type during flexion and extension, the other during axial rotation.

During **flexion and extension** (fig. 120) the patella moves in sagittal plane. Starting from its position in extension (A) it recedes while moving along *the arc of a circle* with centre at the tibial tuberosity (O) and radius equal to the length of the ligamentum patellae. During this movement *it is tilted on itself by an angle of about* 35° in such a way that its deep surface, which faced posteriorly initially, now looks posteriorly and inferiorly in full flexion (B). Therefore it also undergoes a movement of **circumferential displacement** relative to the tibia. This backward movement of the patella is the result of the *two following mechanisms*:

posterior displacement (D) of the point of contact between femoral and tibial condyles;

the shortening of the distance (R) separating the patella from the axis of flexion and extension (+).

During **movements of axial rotation** (figs. 121 to 123), the patella moves relative to the tibia in a *frontal plane*. In the **neutral position** (fig. 121) the ligamentum patellae runs slightly obliquely inferiorly and laterally. During **lateral rotation** (fig. 123) the femur is laterally rotated relative to the tibia and this *drags the patella laterally*; the ligamentum patellae now runs obliquely inferiorly and laterally. During **lateral rotation** (fig. 123) the opposite movements occur: the femur *draws the patella medially* so that the ligamentum patellae runs obliquely inferiorly and laterally but with a greater obliquity than in the neutral position.

The displacements of the patella in relation to the tibia are therefore *indispensable* for movement of *flexion and extension* and of *axial rotation*.

It is easy to demonstrate on a mechanical model that *the patella is responsible for the shape of the patellar surface and the anterior aspects of the condyles of the femur*. During its movements the patella is in effect attached to the tibia by the ligamentum patellae and to the femur by the femoropatellar fibres (p. 104). During knee flexion, the femoral condyles move on the tibial condyles and the deep surface of the patella, dragged along by its ligamentous attachments, moves along a surface which is *geometrically* equivalent to the anterior profile of the femoral condyles, i.e. *the curve that encompasses the successive positions of the deep surface of the patella*. The anterior profile of the femoral condyles is determined therefore essentially by the mechanical attachments of the patella and their arrangement just as the posterior profile of these condyles depends upon the cruciate ligaments.

We have seen (p. 88) how the condylo-trochlear profile of the distal femur is moulded by the tibia and the patella, which are attached to the femur by the cruciate ligaments and the ligamentum patellae and the medial and lateral retinacula respectively.

Operations displacing the tibial tuberosity anteriorly (Maquet) or medially (Elmslie), alter the relationships between patella and trochlea, in particular the force vector promoting coaptation of the articular surfaces and lateral subluxation. Hence their value in the treatment of **patellar syndromes**.

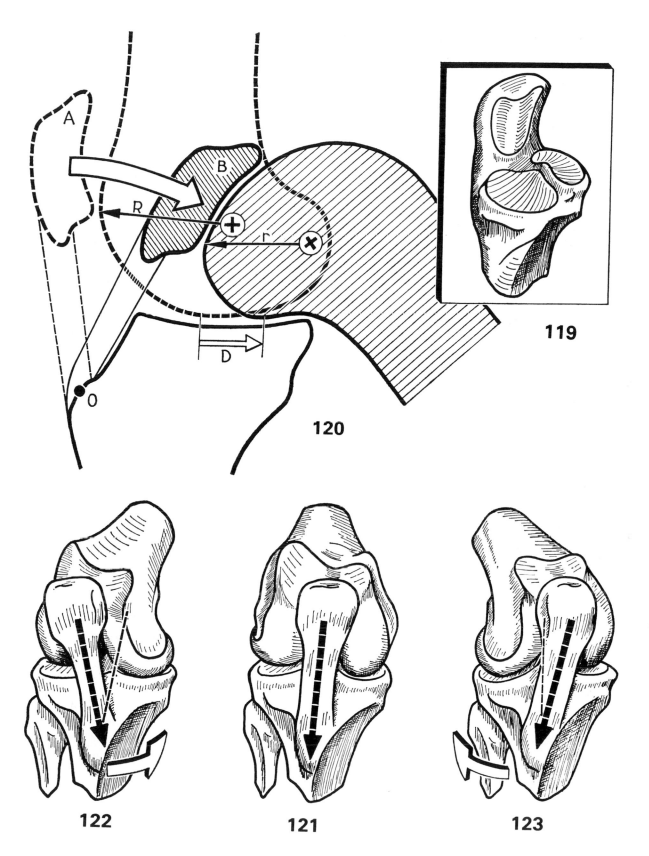

119

120

122

121

123

THE COLLATERAL LIGAMENTS OF THE KNEE

The stability of the knee depends upon the action of *powerful ligaments*, i.e. the cruciate and the collateral ligaments.

The **collateral ligaments** strengthen the articular capsule on its medial and lateral aspects. They are therefore responsible for the transverse stability of the knee during extension.

The medial collateral ligament (fig. 124) runs from the medial aspect of the medial femoral condyle to the upper end of the tibia (MCL):

its femoral insertion lies on the postero-superior aspect of the condyle, *posterior and superior to the line of the centres of curvature* (xx') *of the condyle* (p. 80);

it is attached to the medial aspect of the tibia *posterior to the insertions of the three medial tibial muscles* (sartorius, gracilis and semimembranosus);

its anterior fibres are separate from those of the capsule but its posterior fibres blend intimately with those of the capsule *at the medial border of the medial meniscus*;

it runs obliquely inferiorly and anteriorly, i.e. it crosses in space the direction of the lateral collateral ligament (arrow A).

The lateral collateral ligament (fig. 125) runs from the outer surface of the lateral condyle to the head of the fibula (LCL):

it is attached to the femur *superior and posterior to the line of the centres of curvature* (yy') *of the lateral condyle*;

it is attached to the *fibular head* anterior to its styloid process and deep to the insertion of the biceps;

it is *free of the capsule* along its entire course;

it *runs obliquely inferiorly and posteriorly* and so crosses in space the direction of the medial collateral ligament (arrow B).

In diagrams (figs. 124 and 125) the *meniscopatellar fibres* are seen (1 and 2) as well as the *alar folds* (3 and 4), which keep the patella against the femur.

The collateral ligaments become taut during extension (figs. 126 and 128) and **slackened during flexion** (figs. 127 and 129). Figures 126 and 127 show the difference (d) in length of the medial collateral ligament in the positions of extension and flexion; the change in the obliquity of its postero-inferior course is also shown. Figures 128 and 129 show the same changes in the lateral collateral ligament, i.e. change in length (e) and change in obliquity of its course; from extension to flexion, the direction of the ligament changes from oblique *inferiorly and posteriorly to oblique inferiorly and slightly anteriorly*.

The change in tension in the ligaments can be easily illustrated by **a mechanical model** (fig. 130). A wedge C slides from position 1 to position 2 on a block of wood B and fits into a strap ab attached to the block at a. When c moves from 1 to 2 the strap, which is taken to be elastic, is stretched and assumes a new length ab' so that the difference in length e corresponds to the difference in the thickness of the wedge between points 1 and 2.

In the knee, as extension proceeds, the femoral condyle slides like a wedge between the tibial condyle and the upper attachment of the collateral ligament: the condyle behaves like a wedge because its *radius of curvature increases progressively postero-anteriorly*, while the collateral ligaments are attached *within the concavity of the line joining its centres of curvature*. Flexion at 30° relaxes the collateral ligaments and is the position of immobilisation following repair of these ligaments.

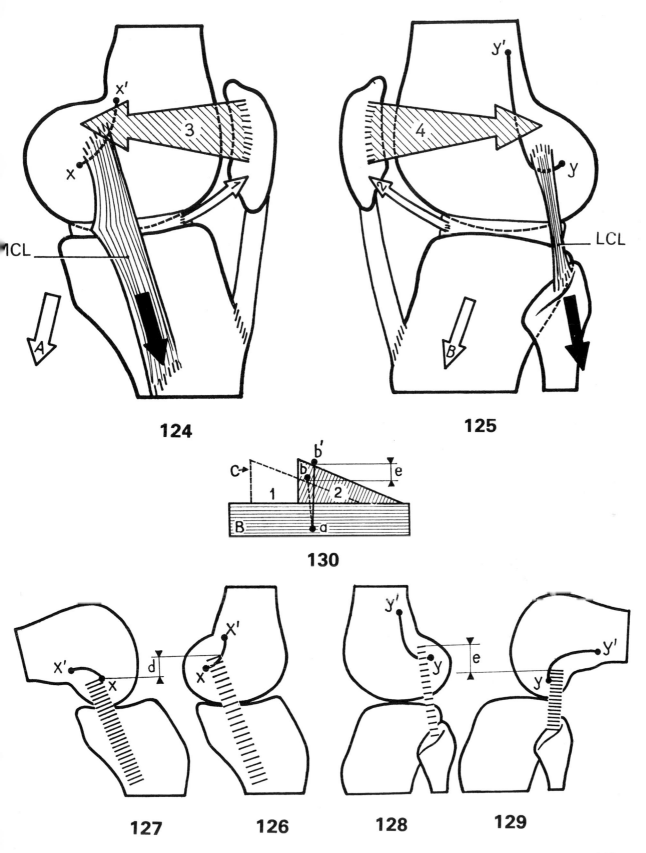

MCL

3

A

124

y'

4

LCL

B

125

c→

b'

b'

e

1

2

B

a

130

x'

x'

d

x

x

127

126

y'

y

e

y'

y

128

129

105

THE TRANSVERSE STABILITY OF THE KNEE

The knee is subjected to considerable side-to-side stresses which are reflected in *the structure of the bony extremities* (fig. 131). As in the upper end of the femur, various bony trabeculae are present along the *lines of the mechanical stresses*:

The distal end of the femur contains *two main sets of trabeculae*: the one runs from the *cortical bone of the inner surface* of the femur and fans out into the ipsilateral condyle (compression forces) and into the contralateral condyle (traction forces); the other runs from *the cortical bone of the lateral surface* and fans out in a corresponding fashion. Another system of trabeculae runs horizontally to unite the two condyles.

The proximal end of the tibia has a similar set of trabeculae which start from the cortical bone of the medial and lateral surfaces and radiate out respectively into the ipsilateral condyle (compression forces) and into the contralateral condyle (traction forces). These two condyles are united by horizontal trabeculae.

Since the femoral axis runs inferiorly and *medially*, the force (F) applied to the superior aspect of the tibia is not strictly vertical (fig. 132) and can therefore be resolved into a vertical component (v) and a transverse component (t), which points horizontally and medially. This component (t) tends to tilt the joint medially and *exaggerate the physiological valgus* by widening the interspace medially (a). the medial ligaments normally prevent such a dislocation.

This transverse component (t) is greater the more marked the physiological valgus (fig. 133). For a force F_2 corresponding to a state of genu valgum (angle of valgus = 160°) the transverse component (t) is twice as great as it is with a normal degree of valgus (170°: F_1 and t_1). Hence *the more marked the genu valgum, the greater its tendency to increase in severity and the greater the demands imposed on the medial ligaments.*

During violent injuries involving the medial and lateral aspects of the knee the upper end of the tibia can be fractured. If the **force is applied to the medial aspect of the knee** (fig. 134), it tends to *straighten out the physiological valgus* and produces first a *fracture-dislocation of the medial tibial condyle* (1) and, if the force is strong enough, a *rupture of the lateral collateral ligament* (2). If the ligament snaps straight away the tibia escapes fracture.

When the **force is applied to the lateral aspect of the knee** (fig. 135), e.g. by the bumper of a car, the lateral femoral condyle is first of all slightly displaced medially and then becomes impacted into the lateral tibial condyle and eventually splits the cortical bone of the lateral aspect of the tibial condyle. This produces a *mixed type of fracture* of the lateral tibial condyle (i.e. impaction-dislocation).

106

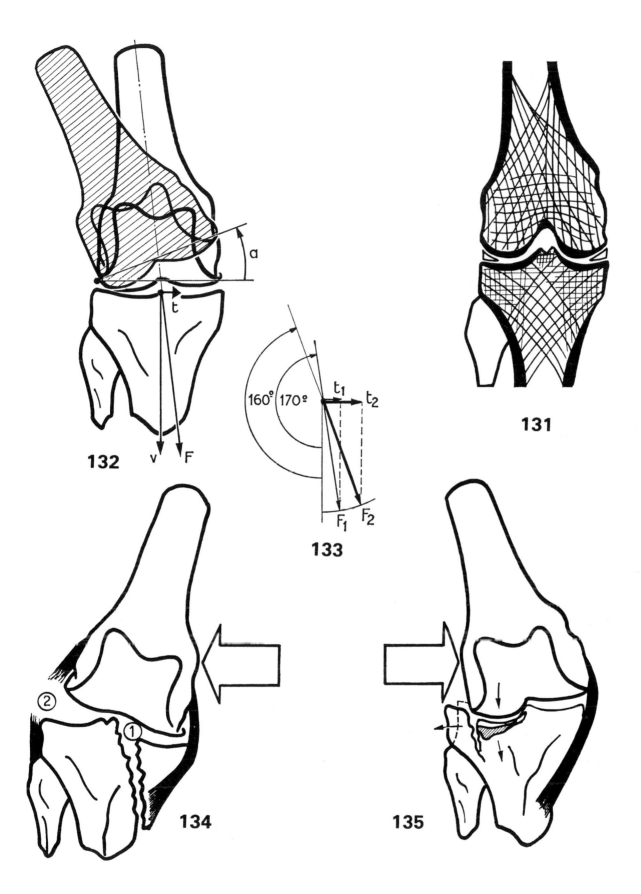

132

α

t

v F

133

160° 170°

t₁ t₂

F₁ F₂

131

134

②

①

135

THE TRANSVERSE STABILITY OF THE KNEE—(*Continued*)

During walking and running the knee is continually subjected to side-to-side stresses. In certain postures the body is in a **state of imbalance, being tilted medially** relative to the supporting knee (fig. 136), this *tends to exaggerate the physiological valgus* and to open out the interspace of the joint *medially*. If the stress is too severe *the medial collateral ligament is torn* (fig. 137) leading to a **severe sprain of the medial collateral ligament** (it must be stressed that this severe degree of sprain does not result purely from the state of imbalance and requires in addition the application of a strong force).

When the body is in the **other state of imbalance, i.e. tilted laterally** relative to the supporting knee (fig. 138) this *tends to straighten out the physiological valgus* and to open out the interspace of the joint *laterally*. If a violent force is applied to the medial aspect of the knee the lateral collateral ligament can be torn as a result, i.e. the **severe sprain of the lateral collateral ligament** (fig. 139).

When the knee is severely sprained, abnormal side-to-side movements can be demonstrated about an anteroposterior axis. For their demonstration the knee must be completely extended or slightly flexed, and these movements must always be compared with those obtained in the other healthy knee.

When the knee is **extended** (fig. 141) or, one might say, hyperextended by the sheer weight of the limb:

any **lateral movement** or valgus indicates combined rupture of the medial collateral ligament (fig. 137) and of the fibro-ligamentous structures lying posteriorly, i.e. the medial condylar plate and the insertion of the medial meniscus into the capsule.

any **medial movement** or varus indicates combined rupture of the lateral collateral ligament (fig. 38) and of the fibroligamentous structures lying posteriorly, essentially the shell of the lateral condylar plate.

When the knee is **flexed at 10°** (fig. 142) these movements indicate isolated rupture of the medial or lateral collateral ligament, since the condyles are slackened in early flexion. It is impossible to be certain in what position a radiograph was taken and so one cannot diagnostically rely on the presence of a gaping joint-space medially in the forced valgus position or laterally in the forced varus position.

In reality it is very difficult to examine a painful knee successfully and it is imperative to do so **under general anaesthesia**.

A severe sprain of the ligaments impairs the stability of the knee. In fact, when the lateral collateral ligament is torn the knee cannot resist the lateral stresses to which it is continually subjected (figs. 136 and 138).

When violent side-to-side stresses are applied during walking or running the collateral ligaments are not the only structures available to stabilise the knee; they are assisted by the *muscles* which form *true active ligaments* and play a vital part in securing the stability of the joint (fig. 140).

The lateral collateral ligament (LCL) is powerfully assisted by the *iliotibial tract* (1), which is tightened by the *tensor fasciae latae* whose contraction is shown in figure 138.

The medial collateral ligament (MCL) is likewise assisted by contraction of *the medial tibial muscles*, i.e. sartorius (2), semitendinosus (3), gracilis (4) whose contraction is shown in action figure 136.

The collateral ligaments are therefore 'lined' by thick muscle tendons. They are also assisted as powerfully by the **quadriceps** with its *straight* (S) and *cruciate* (C) fibres forming a predominantly fibrous canopy for the anterior aspect of the joint. The straight fibres prevent the opening out of the interspace of the joint on the same side, while the cruciate fibres prevent its opening out on the other side. Therefore each vastus muscle, by virtue of its two types of fibres of insertion, influences the stability of the knee both on its medial and lateral aspects. This highlights the significance of the quadriceps in **maintaining the stability of the knee** as well as the abnormal positions of the knee resulting from atrophy of the quadriceps (i.e. 'the knee that gives way').

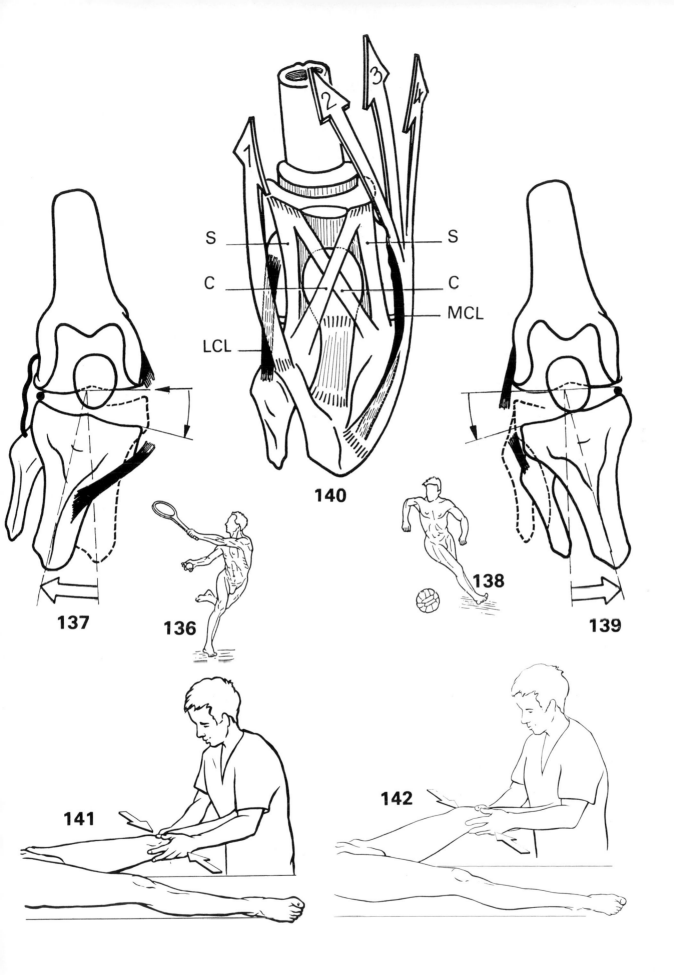

S

C

LCL

S

C

MCL

140

137

136

138

139

141

142

ANTEROPOSTERIOR STABILITY OF THE KNEE

The mechanism of stabilisation of the joint varies according to whether it is slightly flexed or hyperextended.

When **the knee is straight and very slightly flexed** (fig. 143), the force exerted by the body weight acts *behind the flexion and extension axis* of the knee and so the knee tends to flex further unless prevented by contraction of the quadriceps. Therefore in this position the *quadriceps is essential for the maintenance of the erect posture*. On the other hand, if the knee is **hyperextended** (fig. 144) the natural tendency for this hyperextension to increase is soon checked by the capsule and the related ligaments posteriorly (shown in black): *so this erect posture can be maintained without the quadriceps*. This explains why during paralysis of the quadriceps, the state of genu recurvatum is voluntarily exaggerated to allow the patient to stand and even to walk.

When the knee is hyperextended (fig. 145) the axis of the thigh runs obliquely inferiorly and posteriorly and the active force (f) can be resolved into a vertical vector (v) representing the body weight acting on the leg, and a horizontal vector (h), which points posteriorly and so tends to accentuate hyperextension. The more oblique posteriorly is the direction of the force (f), the greater is the vector (h) and the more stretched are the posterior ligaments. Therefore if the genu recurvatum is too severe, these ligaments are eventually overstretched and a vicious circle is set up with further accentuation of the genu recurvatum.

Though limitation of hyperextension of the knee is not provided by bony contact, as with the elbow, yet it is no less efficient (fig. 146) and depends essentially on the capsule and the related ligaments and secondarily on the periarticular muscles.

The capsule and its related ligaments consist of:

the posterior capsular ligament (fig. 147);

the collateral ligaments and the posterior cruciate ligament (fig. 148).

The posterior aspect of the capsule (fig. 147) is strengthened by powerful fibrous bands. On either side, in relation to the femoral condyles, the capsule is thickened to form the 'condylar plates' (1), which give attachment to the heads of the gastrocnemius on their deep surfaces. From the styloid process of the fibula radiates a fan-shaped ligament, *the arcuate ligament of the knee*, which contains two bands:

the *lateral band* or the short lateral ligament of Valois, which blends with the lateral 'condylar plate' (2) and its sesamoid bone (3);

the *medial band* radiates medially and its lowermost (4) fibres from the *popliteal tunnel*, which straddles the popliteus tendon as it goes into the capsule (white arrow).

On the medial side the posterior aspect of the capsule is reinforced by the *oblique popliteal ligament* (5), which is formed by recurrent fibres of the semimembranosus tendon (6) and fans out to be inserted into the lateral 'condylar plate'.

All these ligamentous structures of the posterior aspect of the joint are stretched during hyperextension (fig. 148), especially the *'condylar plates'* (1). As shown previously, during extension the *lateral* (7) and *medial* (8) *collateral ligaments* are stretched. *The posterior cruciate ligament* (9) is also stretched during extension. It is easy to establish that during hyperextension the upper attachments (A, B, C) of these structures move anteriorly about the point O as centre.

Finally the **flexor muscles** (fig. 149) play an *active* part in limiting extension: the *three medial tibial muscles* (10), which course behind the medial femoral condyle; the biceps (11) and also the two heads of the *gastrocnemius* (12). They check extension insofar as they are stretched by dorsiflexion of the ankle.

110

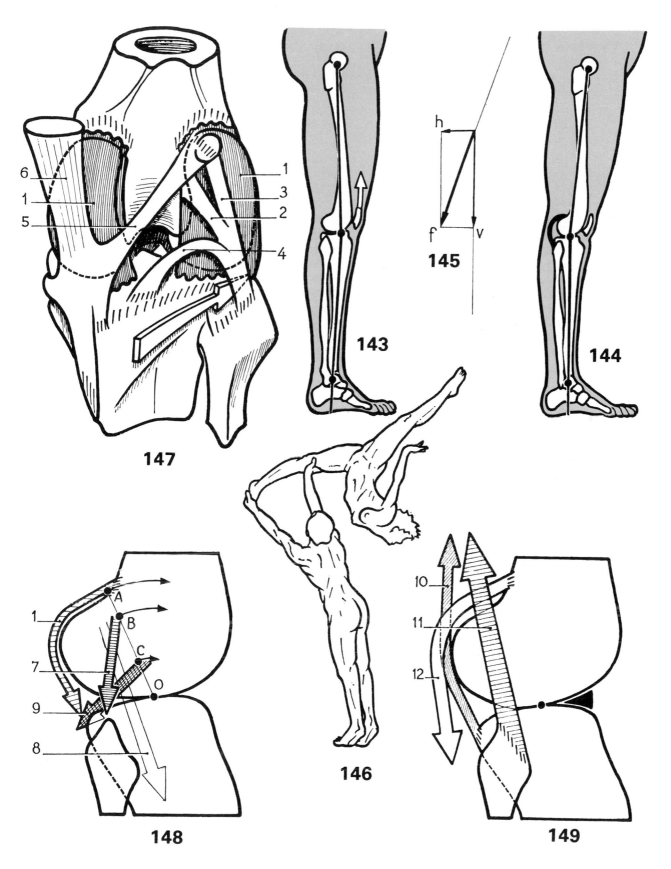

147

143

145

144

146

148

149

111

THE PERIARTICULAR DEFENCE SYSTEM OF THE KNEE

The various capsular and ligamentous structures, so far described analytically, constitute an integrated whole, i.e. the **periarticular defence system of the knee** (fig. 150).

A transverse section of the knee through the joint space reveals:

medially, the medial tibial condyle (1), with the medial meniscus (2);

laterally, the lateral tibial condyle (3) with the lateral meniscus (4), attached to the medial by the intermeniscal ligament (5);

anteriorly, the patella (6), overhanging the anterior tibial tubercle (7) and the anterior insertion of the anterior cruciate ligament (8);

posteriorly, the posterior insertion of the posterior cruciate ligament (9).

The periarticular defence system of the knee comprises **three major components**: the medial collateral ligament, the lateral collateral ligament and the posterior capsular complex.

the **medial collateral ligament** (10), according to F. Bonnel, can sustain a force of 115 kg/cm^2 and a stretch of 12·5% of its length before rupture.

the **lateral collateral ligament** (11) can sustain a force of 276 kg/cm^2 and a stretch of 19 per cent of its length before rupture. It is thus unexpectedly at once more resistant and more elastic than the medial ligament.

the **posterior capsulo-fibrous complex** consists of the shell of the medial tibial condyle (12), the shell of the lateral condyle (13) with its sesamoid bone or fabella (14), and the oblique posterior ligament (15) and the cruciate ligament (16).

There are four **accessory** fibrotendinous sheets of unequal strength and importance:

the **posteromedial sheet**, lying posterior to the medial collateral ligament, is the most important and comprises:

the most posterior fibres of the medial collateral ligament (10 bis);

the medial border of the medial tibial condyle (12);

two extensions of the semimembranosus tendon (16) i.e. the reflected insertion (17) running inferior to the edge of the medial tibial condyle and the meniscal insertion (18), attached to the posterior edge of the medial meniscus.

the **posterolateral sheet** is clearly less strong than the former, because at this point the lateral meniscus is separated from the capsule and the lateral collateral ligament by the popliteus tendon (19) after it arises from the lateral condyle. The tendon sends a fibrous expansion (20), which tethers the posterior part of the lateral meniscus and is further reinforced by the short fibres of the lateral collateral ligament (21) and the lateral edge of the lateral condyle.

the **anterolateral sheet** is made up of the iliotibial tract (22), which sends an expansion (23) to the lateral border of the patella and of the straight and crossed expansions of the quadriceps tendon, which constitute the lateral compartment of the extensor apparatus.

the **anteromedial sheet** consists of the direct and crossed fibres of the quadriceps tendon (25), reinforced by the tendon of the sartorius (26), attached to the medial border of the patella.

Periarticular muscles also contribute to the defence of the knee joint. By contracting in a manner perfectly synchronised for a particular movement and preconditioned by the cerebral cortex, they prevent mechanical distortions and are indispensable for the ligaments, which can only react passively. The most important of these muscles is the **quadriceps**, which is essential for the stability of the knee. By its strength and its precise coordination it is able up to a point to compensate for ligamentous failure. For any operation to succeed the quadriceps must be in good physical condition. Since it atrophies rapidly and is slow of recovery, it deserves the close attention of surgeon and physiotherapist.

Laterally lies the iliotibial tract (22), which should be considered as the terminal tendon of the **glutei**. Posteromedially lie the semimebranosus (26), the sartorius (27), the gracilis (28) and the semitendinosus (29). Posterolaterally are found two muscles: the popliteus (19), whose peculiar functions will be discussed later, and the biceps femoris (30), whose strong tendon reinforces the lateral collateral ligament.

Posteriorly lies the **gastrocnemius**, which is attached to the femoral condyles. The tendinous insertion of its medial head (31) crosses the tendon of the semimembranosus with an intervening bursa, which is often connected with the joint cavity. The tendinous insertion of its lateral head (33) also crosses the tendon of the biceps but there is no intervening bursa.

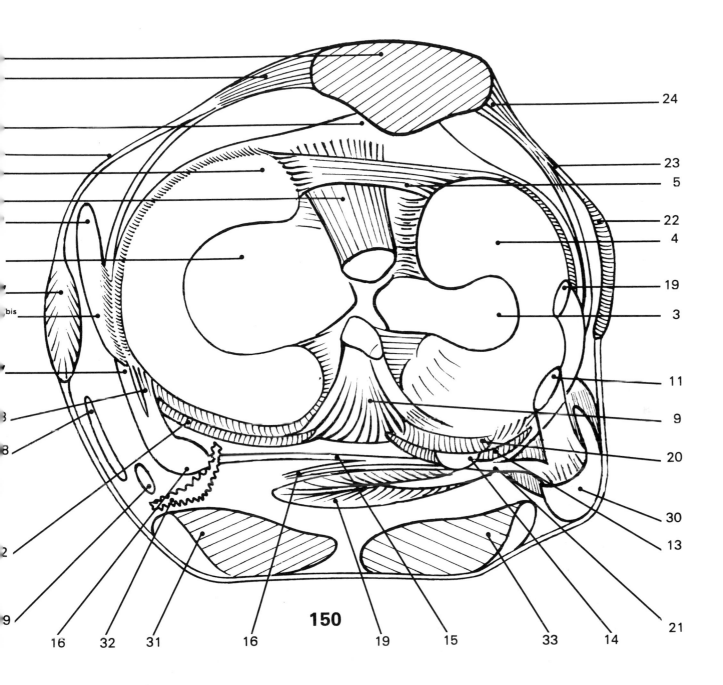

24

23

5

22

4

19

3

11

9

20

30

13

21

bis

150

16   32   31   16   19   15   33   14

113

THE CRUCIATE LIGAMENTS OF THE KNEE

When the joint is opened anteriorly (fig. 151, according to Rouvière) it becomes obvious that the cruciate ligaments lie in **the centre of the joint** being largely contained within the intercondylar notch.

The first ligament to be seen is the **anterior cruciate ligament** (1), which is attached (fig. 152 (5), according to Rouvière) to the anterior intercondylar fossa of the tibia, along the edge of the medial condyle and between the insertion of the anterior horn of the medial meniscus anteriorly (7) and that of the lateral meniscus (8) posteriorly (see also fig. 73). *It runs obliquely superiorly and laterally* and is attached above (1) (fig. 153, according to Rouvière), to a narrow patch on the internal aspect of the lateral condyle of the femur which extends vertically above and along the edge of the articular cartilage (fig. 73). The ligament has a *more anterior attachment to the tibia* and *a more lateral attachment to the femur* than its fellow; hence the name anterolateral ligament is more apposite.

It consists of three bands:

the **anteromedial** band, the longest, most superficial and most prone to injury;

the **posterolateral** band, lying deep to the former and unaffected in partial tears of the ligament;

the **intermediate** band.

As a whole, the ligament is twisted on itself so that its most anterior tibial fibres are inserted into the femur the most anteriorly and inferiorly and its most posterior tibial fibres are inserted the most superiorly into the femur. As a result, the fibres vary in length depending on their location and, according to Bonnel, their mean lengths range from 1·85 to 3·35 cm.

In the depths of the intercondylar notch behind the anterior cruciate can be seen (fig. 151) **the posterior cruciate ligament** (2). It is attached (fig. 152) to the posterior part of the posterior intercondylar fossa of the tibia, overlapping (according to Rouvière, figs. 153 and 154) the posterior rim of the upper surface of the tibia (fig. 73). Its *tibial insertion* (fig. 152) is therefore placed well posterior to the insertion of the posterior horns of the lateral (9) and medial menisci (10). The ligament *runs obliquely medially, anteriorly and superiorly* (fig. 154: knee flexed 90°) to be inserted (2) into the depths of the intercondylar notch (fig. 155, according to Rouvière) and also to a patch on the edge of the lateral surface of the medial condyle along the line of the articular cartilage (fig. 76). Therefore this ligament has a *more posterior attachment to the tibia* and *a more medial attachment to the femur* than its fellow; hence the more suitable name of the posteromedial ligament.

It comprises four bands:

the **posterolateral** band, inserted the most posteriorly into the tibia and the most laterally into the femur;

the **anteromedial** band, inserted the most anteriorly into the tibia and the most medially into the femur;

the **anterior band of Humphrey**, often absent;

the **menisco-femoral ligament of Wrisberg** (3), which is attached to the posterior horn of the lateral meniscus (figs. 152 and 153), clings to the anterior surface (usually) of the main ligament (fig. 151) and runs with it to a common insertion into the lateral surface of the medial condyle. Occasionally a *similar ligament is present in relation to the medial meniscus* (fig. 152); a few fibres (12) of the anterior cruciate are inserted into the anterior horn of the medial meniscus near the insertion of the transverse ligament (11).

The cruciate ligaments *touch each other* (fig. 155: the cruciates have been sectioned near their femoral end) on their axial borders, with the anterior running lateral to the posterior ligament. They do not lie free within the joint cavity but are *lined by synovium* and they have important relations with the capsule.

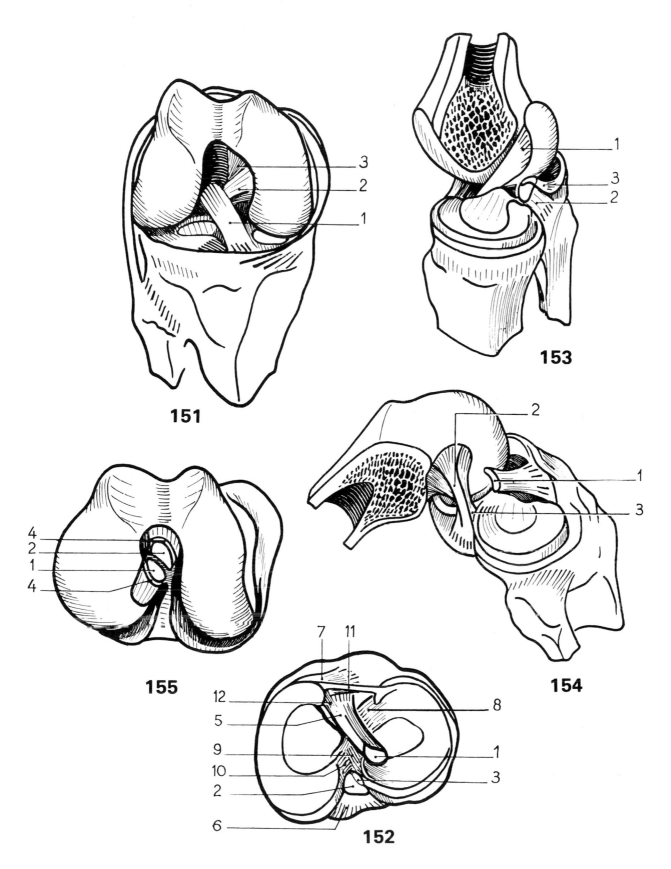

151

153

155

154

152

115

RELATIONS OF THE CAPSULE AND THE CRUCIATE LIGAMENTS

The cruciates are so intimately related to the capsule that they can be considered as **actual thickenings of the capsule** and, as such, as integral parts of the capsule. It has been shown (p. 88) how the capsule dips into the intercondylar notch to form a double-layered partition along the axis of the joint. It was said earlier, for the sake of convenience, that, to a first approximation, the attachment of the capsule (fig. 156) was such as to make the tibial insertions of the cruciates extracapsular. In fact, the *capsular attachment passes through the attachments* of the cruciates and the thickenings of the capsule, formed by the cruciates, simply stand out on its external surface, i.e. between the two layers of the partition.

Figure 157 (seen from behind and inside: after removal of the medial condyle and section of part of the capsule) shows the **anterior cruciate ligament** clearly applied to the external layer of the capsular partition (the posterior cruciate is not included).

Figure 158 (seen from behind and outside; same as fig. 157) shows the **posterior cruciate** applied to the internal layer of the capsular partition.

Note that all the fibres of the cruciates do not have the same length or the same direction (fig. 159); therefore during movements of the knee they are not all stretched at the same time (p. 120).

These diagrams also illustrate the 'condylar plates', left untouched over the medial condyle (fig. 158) and partially resected over the lateral condyle (fig. 157).

A coronal section (fig. 156), passing through the posterior part of the condyles, illustrates the division of the joint cavity (femur and tibia have been artificially pulled apart):

In the middle the capsular partition, thickened by the cruciate ligaments, divides the cavity into a lateral and a medial compartment, this partition is extended anteriorly by the infrapatellar pad (p. 90); each compartment is in turn divided into two storeys by the meniscus, the upper or *suprameniscal* storey corresponding to the line of contact between femur and meniscus, and the lower or *inframeniscal* storey corresponding to the line of contact between tibia and meniscus.

It is the presence of the cruciate ligaments that profoundly alters the structure of this hinge-joint (the term 'bicondylar joint' is meaningless mechanically). The anterior cruciate (fig. 159) from its initial neutral position (1) starts by lying down horizontally (2) on the tibial plateau during flexion to 45°–50° and then climbs to its highest point (3) during extreme flexion. As it moves down towards the tibia, it lodges itself in the interspinal groove, as if it had 'sawn' through the tibial spines like a bread-knife (inset). In its motion during extension (A) to extreme flexion (B) the posterior cruciate ligament (fig. 160) sweeps a much wider sector (with an angle of nearly 60°) than the anterior cruciate and it 'carves' in the femur the intercondylar notch, which separates the two sides of the physiological pulley formed by the condyles.

116

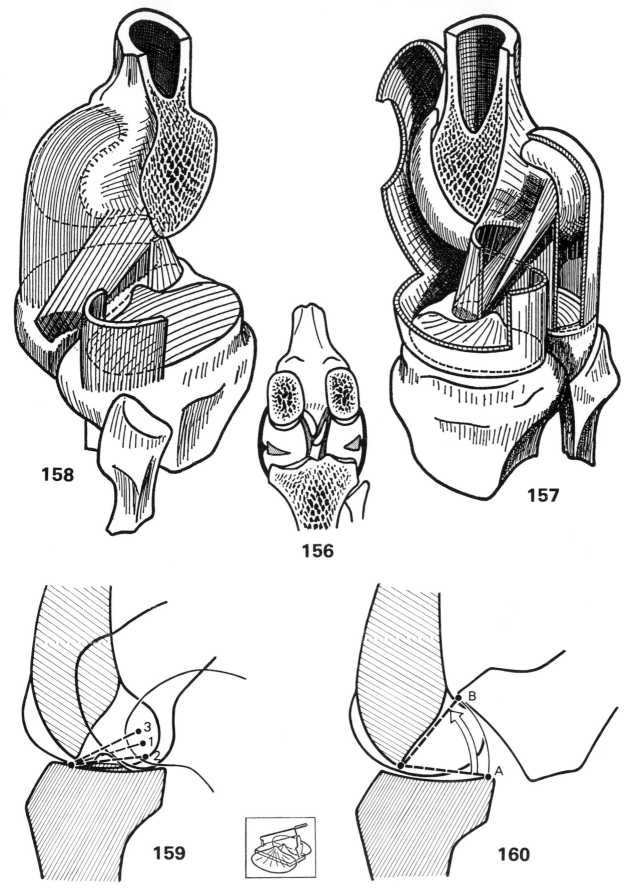

158

156

157

159

160

THE DIRECTION OF THE CRUCIATE LIGAMENTS

Seen in perspective (fig. 161), these ligaments appear to be in fact **crossed in space**. In the *sagittal* plane (fig. 162) they are crossed, with the anterior cruciate (AC) running obliquely superiorly and *posteriorly* and the posterior cruciate (PC) running superiorly and *anteriorly*. They are also crossed in the *frontal* plane (fig. 163, posterior view) as their tibial attachments (black dots) lie on the anteroposterior axis of the joint (arrow S) while their femoral insertions are 1·7 cm. apart. Thus the posterior cruciate runs obliquely superiorly and *medially* and the anterior obliquely superiorly and *laterally*. In the horizontal plane, by contrast (fig. 185), they run *parallel* to each other and are in contact at their axial borders.

The cruciates not only cross each other in space but also the *ipsilateral collateral ligament*: thus the anterior ligament and the lateral collateral ligament are crossed (fig. 165) and the posterior ligament and the medial collateral ligament are also crossed (fig. 166). Therefore each of these ligaments alternates with its immediate neighbour as regards the obliquity of its course (when taken in order mediolaterally or lateromedially).

The cruciate ligaments **do not have the same angle of inclination** (fig. 162). Thus in full extension the anterior cruciate (AC) is more vertical while the posterior cruciate (PC) is more horizontal. Their femoral insertions show a similar difference: thus the insertion of the posterior cruciate is horizontal (b) while that of the anterior cruciate is vertical (a).

When the knee is flexed (fig. 164), the posterior cruciate, which lies flat horizontally during extension, rears itself up vertically, sweeping a 60° angle with respect to the tibia, while the anterior cruciate is raised only very slightly.

The length ratio of the cruciate ligaments shows individual variations, but is typical of each knee insofar as it is one of the determinants of the shape of the condyles, as demonstrated earlier.

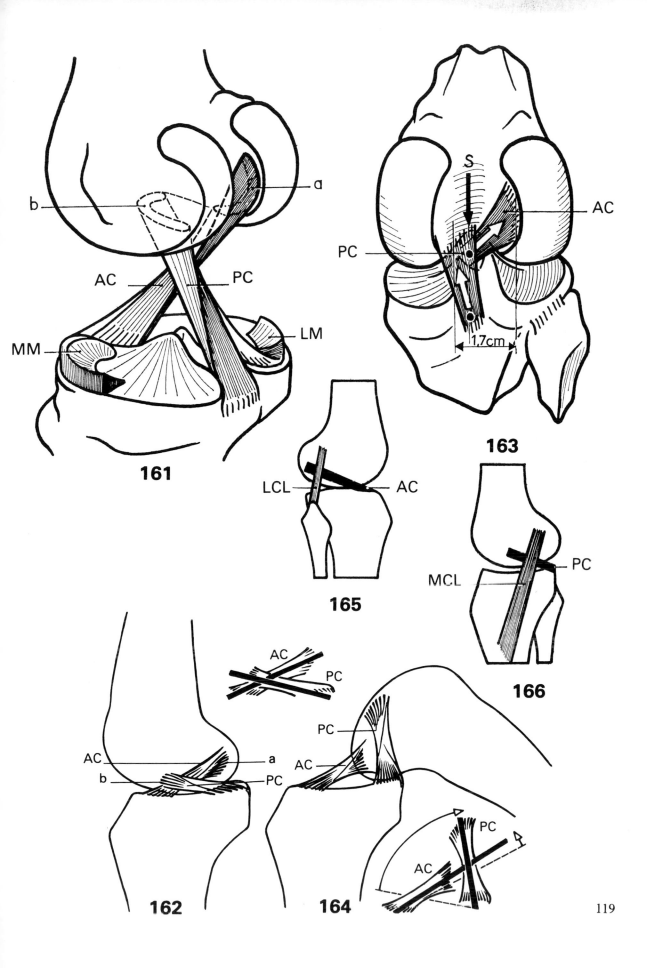

161

163

165

166

162

164

119

THE MECHANICAL ROLE OF THE CRUCIATE LIGAMENTS

It is customary to reduce the cruciate ligaments to linear *cords* with *pointline* attachments. This is true as a first approximation and has the advantage of helping one to understand the general actions of the ligaments but it fails to reveal their **functional subtleties**. For this purpose three factors must be taken into account:

1. THE THICKNESS TO THE LIGAMENT

The thickness and volume of a ligament are directly proportional to its strength and inversely proportional to its elasticity. Each fibre can be considered as a small spring.

2. THE STRUCTURE OF THE LIGAMENT

Because of the size of its attachments the fibres do not have the same length, with the **important consequence** that the fibres are not called into action simultaneously. As with muscular fibres, there is **fibre recruitment** during movements and, as a result, the strength and elasticity of the ligament are variable.

3. THE SIZE AND DIRECTION OF ITS ATTACHMENTS

Moreover the fibres are *not always parallel* but are often *twisted*, because the lines linking their attachment points are not parallel but more often oblique or perpendicular to one another. Also the relative orientation of the attachments varies during movements, contributing to fibre recruitment and modifying the action of the ligament as a whole. These changes in the direction of the ligament take place not only in the sagittal plane but in **all three planes**, accounting for its complex and simultaneous actions on the anteroposterior, lateral and rotational stability of the knee.

Thus the geometry of the cruciate ligaments determines the shape of femoral condyles and trochlea in *all three planes of space*.

As a whole, the cruciate ligaments ensure the **anteroposterior stability** of the knee and allow **hinge-like movements** to occur while keeping the articular surfaces together.

Their role can be illustrated by an easily constructed *mechanical model* (fig. 167). Two planks A and B (seen in cross-section) are attached by two ribbons (ab and cd) linking the opposite ends of the planes. They can thus move with respect to each other about two hinges. The points a and b can be superimposed on c and d respectively but *there can be no sliding movements*.

The cruciate ligaments resemble the ribbons, except that there are not two hinges but a series of hinges lying along the curve of the condyle. As in the model anteroposterior sliding is impossible.

In the small diagrams on the next two pages the cruciate ligaments are represented by straight lines (anterior = ab and posterior = cd). In the larger diagrams they are represented by their peripheral and middle fibres with their lines of attachment.

Starting from *the neutral position* (fig. 168) or from slight flexion at 30° (fig. 169), when the cruciates are stretched to the same degree, flexion causes tilting of the femoral 'plank' cb (fig. 170), while the posterior ligament cd is straightened and the anterior ligament ab becomes horizontal. As seen on the more detailed diagram (fig. 171), flexion to 60° has but little effect on the degree of tension in the ligaments.

120

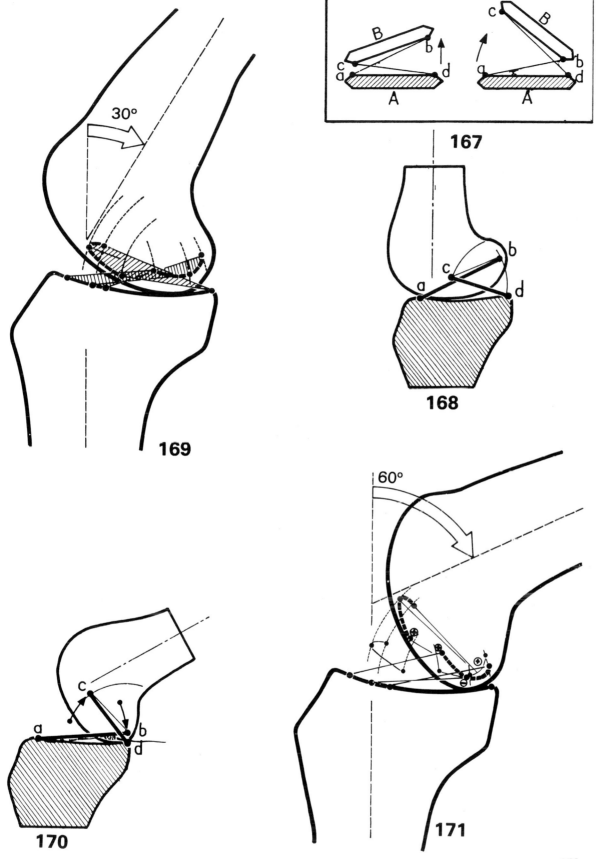

167

168

169

170

171

121

THE MECHANICAL ROLE OF THE CRUCIATE LIGAMENTS—(*Continued*)

When flexion increases to 90° (fig. 172) and then to 120° (fig. 173), the posterior cruciate rears itself up vertically and is proportionately more stretched than the anterior cruciate. As seen in the more detailed diagram (fig. 174), the middle and inferior fibres of the anterior cruciate are relaxed (−) while only the anterosuperior fibres are stretched (+) and vice versa for the posterior cruciate. **The posterior cruciate is stretched during flexion.**

During extension and hyperextension (fig. 175) from the neutral position (figs. 176 and 177), all the fibres of the anterior cruciate are stretched (+), while only the posterosuperior fibres of the posterior ligament are stretched (+). Furthermore, during hyperextension (fig. 178), the floor of the intercondylar fossa c hits the anterior cruciate and stretches it in the manner of a trestle. **The anterior cruciate is stretched during extension and helps to check hyperextension.**

F. Bonnel has recently confirmed these ideas, first enunciated by Strasser (1917), on the basis of a mechanical model. But a more refined mechanical analysis also supports Roud (1913), who stated that the cruciates were always partly under tension as a result of the unequal lengths of their fibres. As is often the case in biomechanics, two apparently contradictory ideas are not mutually exclusive.

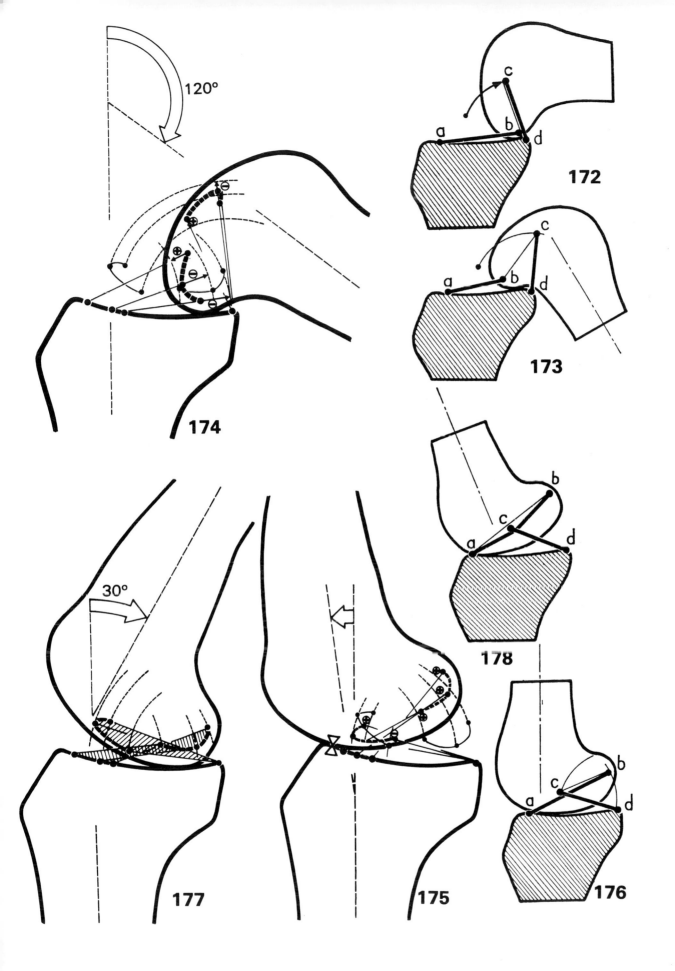

120°

172

173

174

30°

178

177

175

176

THE MECHANICAL ROLE OF THE CRUCIATE LIGAMENTS—(*Continued*)

We have seen that the femoral condyles (p. 84) roll and slide on the tibial plateau. It is easy to visualize the rolling movements but the question arises how does any *sliding* occur in such a tightly interlocked joint. It is **actively** produced by the extensors, which pull the tibia anteriorly under the femur during extension (p. 136) and, conversely, by the flexors, which cause the tibial plateau to slide posteriorly during flexion. But, when these movements are studied on the skeleton, the **passive** role played by the cruciate ligaments assumes even greater significance. *The cruciates pull back the femoral condyles and cause them to slide on the tibial plateau in the direction opposite to their rolling movement.*

Starting (fig. 179) from extension (I), if the condyle rolled without sliding, it should recede to position (II) and the femoral insertion b of the anterior cruciate ab should hit b' after covering the theoretical distance bb'. This situation, illustrated in figure 108 (p. 97), leads to damage of the posterior horn of the medial meniscus. But point b can only move along a circle with centre a and radius ab (the ligament being taken as inelastic); thus the real path of b is not bb' but bb'', corresponding to the position (III) of the femoral condyle, lying anterior to position (II) by a distance of e. During flexion the anterior cruciate is called into action and pulls back the condyle anteriorly. It can be said therefore that during flexion **the anterior cruciate ligament causes the femoral condyle to slide anteriorly** while the latter rolls in a posterior direction.

The role of the posterior cruciate during extension can be similarly demonstrated (fig. 180). As it rolls from position (I) to position (II), the condyle is pulled back posteriorly by the posterior cruciate cd and the path of the femoral insertion of the ligament is not cc' but cc'' along a circle with centre d and radius dc. Thus the condyle slides posteriorly over a distance f to reach position (III). *During extension the posterior cruciate ligament causes the femoral condyle to slide posteriorly* while the latter rolls in an anterior direction.

Drawer movements of the tibia under the femur are *abnormal* and can be demonstrated in two positions: 1) with the knee flexed at right angle and 2) with the knee in full extension.

With the knee flexed at right angles (fig. 183) and the patient lying supine on a hard surface, the examiner sits on the foot and keeps it from moving. He then grasps with both hands the superior end of the leg. By *pulling* the leg anteriorly an *anterior drawer* can be demonstrated and vice versa. This demonstration can be achieved with the foot in *neutral position* as well as in *medial* or *lateral rotation*.

The **posterior drawer** (fig. 181) is produced by posterior displacement of the tibia under the femur and is due to rupture of the posterior cruciate. Hence the mnemonic: **posterior drawer = posterior cruciate**.

The **anterior drawer** (fig. 182) is produced by anterior displacement of the tibia under the femur and is due to rupture of the anterior cruciate. Hence, **anterior drawer = anterior cruciate**.

With the knee extended, the examiner supports the posterior aspect of the thigh with one hand, while the other hand, holding the superior end of the leg, attempts to move it anteriorly and posteriorly (the Lachmann-Trillat test). Any movement anteriorly indicates rupture of the anterior cruciate, particularly, according to Bousquet, rupture of the posterolateral fibrotendinous sheet. This test is difficult to perform because of the small range of movement involved.

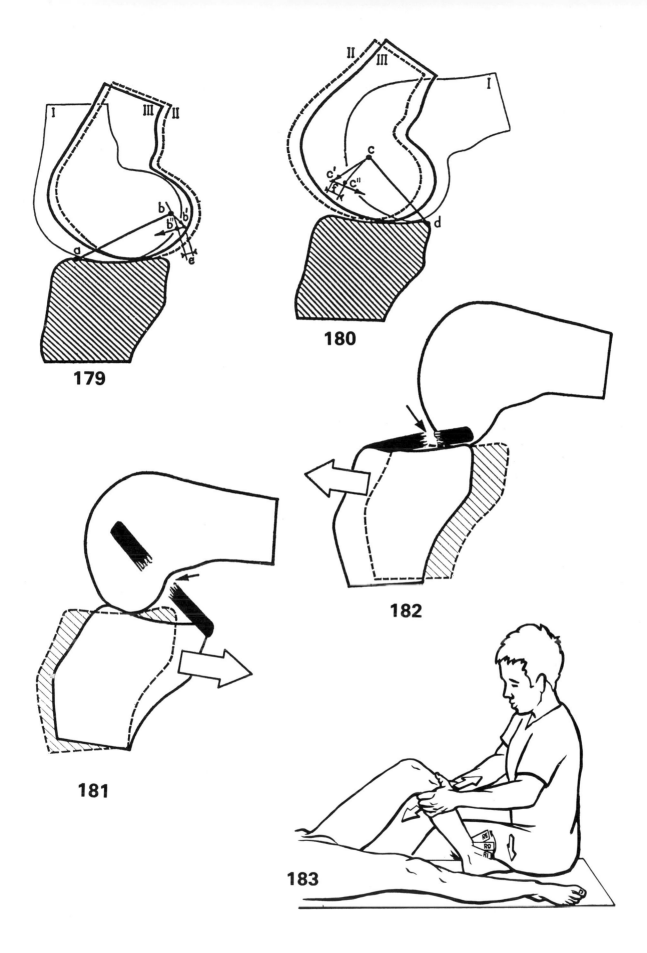

179

180

181

182

183

THE ROTATIONAL STABILITY OF THE KNEE DURING EXTENSION

We already know that movements of axial rotation of the knee can only occur when the knee is flexed. On the other hand, in full extension axial rotation is impossible, being prevented by the taut collateral and cruciate ligaments.

On an anterior view of the knee in neutral rotation (fig. 184: the articular surfaces are widely 'separated' as a result of abnormal 'distensibility' of the ligaments), the *cruciate ligaments are seen to cross each other* and, because of their obliquity (fig. 185: transverse view), they can *wrap themselves round each other*.

During **medial rotation** of the tibia on the femur (fig. 186: frontal view), the direction of the cruciate ligaments is *clearly more crossed* in the frontal plane (inset), while, in the horizontal plane (fig. 187: seen from above), *their axial borders are in contact* (inset). Thus they coil round each other (fig. 188) and *stretch each other* (fig. 189), like the cords of a tourniquet. As a result, *the tibial and femoral surfaces are brought closer together*, effectively preventing medial rotation. At the same time, since the centre of rotation (fig. 187: cross) does not coincide with the centre of the joint but with the medial aspect of the medial tibial spine, medial rotation relaxes the posterior (−) and stretches the anterior (+) cruciate and its fibres attached to the anterior horn of the medial meniscus, which is then pulled back posteriorly.

During **lateral rotation** of the tibia on the femur (fig. 190° anterior view), the ligaments *tend to become parallel* (inset). In the horizontal plane (fig. 191: seen from above) they become *more crossed* but their *axial borders lose contact*. As a result, the 'tourniquet' is relaxed and there is *slight separation* of the articular surfaces (fig. 193). Thus lateral rotation is not checked by stretching of the cruciate ligaments. However, since the centre of rotation fails to coincide with centre of the joint (fig. 191), lateral rotation relaxes the anterior (−) and stretches the posterior (+) cruciate and its fibres inserted into the posterior horn of the lateral meniscus, which is then pulled back anteriorly.

The cruciate ligaments prevent medial rotation of the extended knee.

Medial rotation stretches the anterior cruciate and relaxes the posterior cruciate.

Lateral rotation stretches the posterior cruciate and relaxes the anterior cruciate.

Slocum and Larson have studied in detail the *rotational stability of the flexed knee* in athletes, particularly in football players. When these players turn suddenly towards the side opposite the supporting limb, they subject that knee to violent lateral rotation. The involvement of the *medial part of the articular capsule* under these conditions is demonstrated as follows:

its anterior third is very prone to rupture if the trauma is associated with valgus displacement and lateral rotation while the knee is flexed at 90°;

its posterior third is easily injured when the knee is extended;

its middle third, identical with the deep fibres of the medial collateral ligament, is ruptured when the trauma involves a knee flexed between 30° and 90°.

In addition, if the knee is flexed at right angles or more, the *anterior cruciate* begins to relax during the first 15 to 20 degrees of lateral rotation and then becomes taut again. If lateral rotation is not checked, the ligament may be torn as it wraps itself round the medial surface of the lateral femoral condyle.

Finally, through its capsular connections to the tibia, the *posterior half of the medial meniscus* can by itself prevent lateral rotation of the flexed knee.

In sum, exposure of the flexed knee to graded trauma combining valgus displacement and lateral rotation can cause successively:

rupture of the anterior third of the capsule;

rupture of the medial collateral ligament, deep fibres first and then superficial fibres;

rupture of the anterior cruciate;

detachment of the medial meniscus.

126

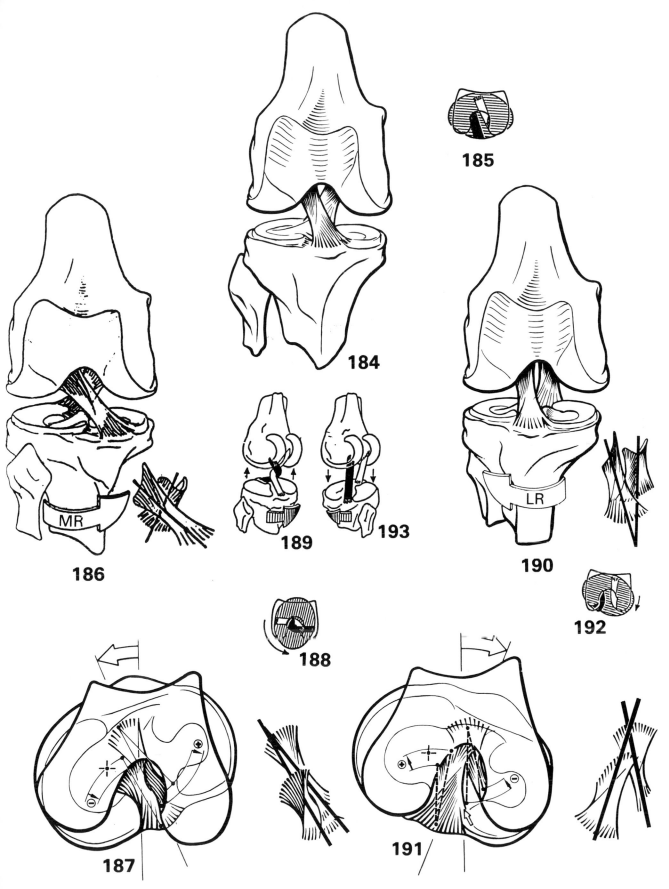

MR = Medial rotation;   LR = Lateral rotation

THE ROTATIONAL STABILITY OF THE KNEE DURING EXTENSION—*(Continued)*

The role of the **collateral ligaments** in ensuring the rotational stability of the knee can be explained by their symmetry.

In the **neutral position** (fig. 194: seen from above with the condyles transparent), the obliquity of the lateral collateral ligament running inferiorly and anteriorly and of the medial collateral ligament running inferiorly and posteriorly causes them to coil round the superior end of the tibia.

Medial rotation (fig. 195) prevents this coiling movement, as the obliquity of these ligaments decreases and they tend to become parallel (fig. 196: posteromedial view with the surfaces separated). As the coiling decreases, the articular surfaces are less strongly apposed by the collateral ligaments (fig. 197), while the opposite effect is achieved by the cruciate ligaments. Thus the 'play' permitted by the relaxation of the collateral is offset by stretching of the cruciates.

Conversely, **lateral rotation** (fig. 198) increases the coiling (fig. 200), which brings the articular surfaces closer together and limits movement. The cruciates are simultaneously relaxed.

Lateral rotation is checked by the collateral ligaments, medial rotation by the cruciate ligaments.

Rotational stability of the extended knee is thus ensured by the collateral and cruciate ligaments.

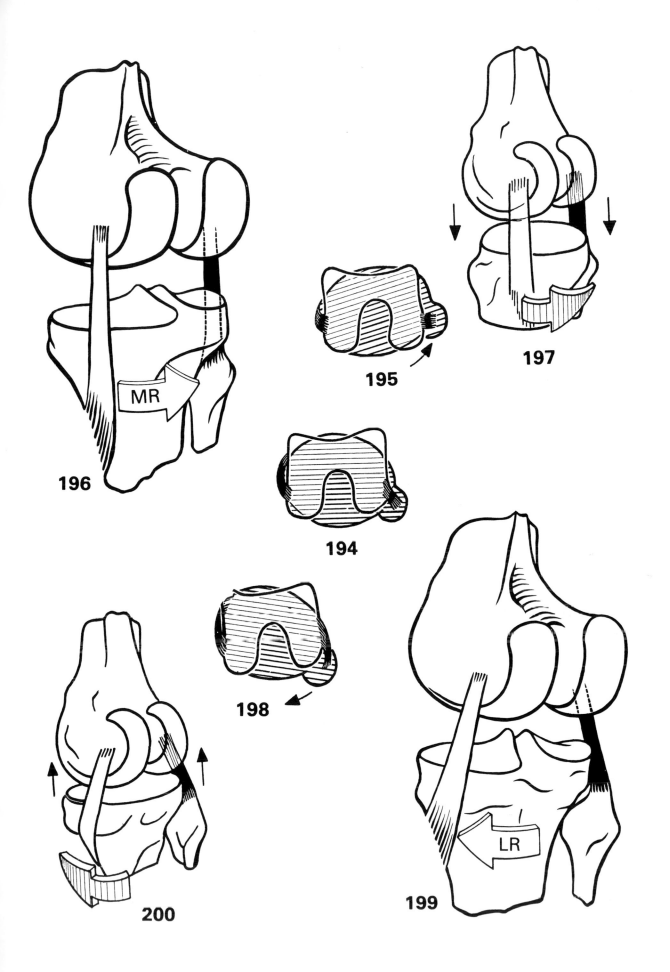

196

195

197

194

198

199

200

MR

LR

DYNAMIC TESTS OF THE KNEE: MEDIAL ROTATION

In addition to static tests of knee stability looking for abnormal transverse and anteroposterior movements, there are now well-recognised *dynamic tests of stability* (or instability), which aim at demonstrating abnormal components of test movements. These tests are so numerous that they need to be classified with emphasis laid on the most important.

It is practical to put these tests into **two groups**:

tests combining valgus displacement and medial rotation;

tests combining valgus displacement and lateral rotation;

The **first group** includes the following:

The **lateral Pivot Shift Test of McIntosh** is the best known and the most widely used. It is performed on a patient lying flat on his back (fig. 201) or at an angle of 45° (fig. 202). In the first case (fig. 201), the examiner uses one hand to hold the foot on its plantar aspect and to produce forced medial rotation; the sheer weight of the limb causes valgus displacement at the knee. In the second case (fig. 202), the examiner's hand holds the foot at the instep with his palm gripping the heel and produces medial rotation by wrist extension. The *neutral position* of the knee is in *extension* (fig. 201); the free hand of the examiner pushes the knee anteriorly to produce *flexion* and inferiorly to increase the degree of *valgus*. During flexion (fig. 202), there is some *resistance to movement* but at 25°–30° flexion there is a sudden *jerk*, as one feels and sees the lateral femoral condyle jump anteriorly on the lateral tibial plateau.

The positive McIntosh test indicates **rupture of the anterior cruciate ligament**. With the knee in extension, medial rotation (fig. 203) shifts the lateral femoral condyle posteriorly on the posterior slope of the convex surface of the lateral tibial plateau and it is held there by the taut fascia lata (FL) and the valgus displacement, both of which keep the articular surfaces in close apposition. As long as the fascia lata lies anterior to the ridge of the convex lateral tibial plateau, the femoral condyle remains fixed in the position of posterior subluxation (PSL). With increasing flexion (fig. 204), the fascia lata moves posterior to the ridge of the lateral tibial plateau, the condyle rides over that ridge and is arrested anteriorly on the anterior slope (2) of the tibial plateau, where it is held in check by the posterior cruciate. It is important to realise that the patient also perceives this sudden jerk.

The *jerk test of Hughston* is the converse of the McIntosh test. It is performed with the patient supine (fig. 205) or lying at an angle of 45° (fig. 206). The difference is that the starting position is at *35° to 40° flexion* and the knee is then extended while a valgus stress is applied to the knee and the foot is medially rotated. The lateral femoral condyle (stippled) initially lies in an 'exaggerated' anterior position, where it is in contact (2) with the anterior slope of the convex lateral tibial plateau. It then jerks posteriorly (PSL) as the anterior cruciate fails to hold it back during extension. Thus a positive Hughston test also indicates rupture of the anterior cruciate.

130

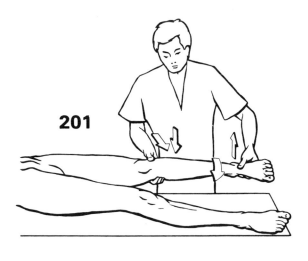

201

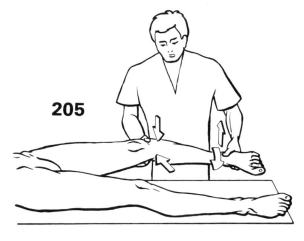

205

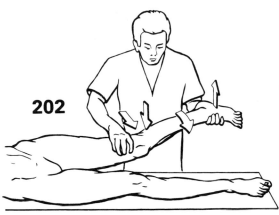

202

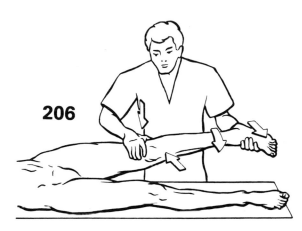

206

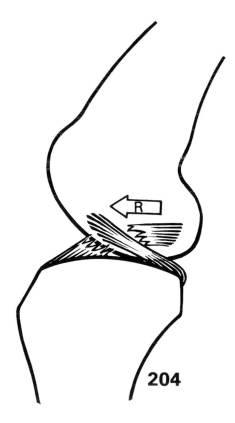

204

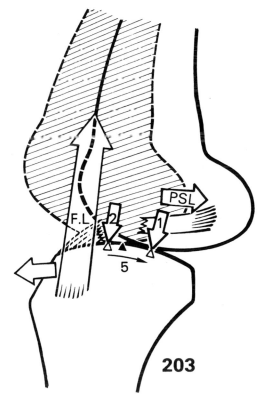

203

DYNAMIC TESTS FOR RUPTURE OF THE ANTERIOR CRUCIATE LIGAMENT

While the McIntosh and the Hughston tests are the most commonly used, the easiest to perform and the most reliable of the dynamic tests, there are three others able to demonstrate rupture of the anterior cruciate.

The **Losee test** (fig. 207) is done with the patient supine. With one hand the examiner supports the heel with the knee *flexed at 30°* and with the other hand he grasps the knee anteriorly with his thumb gripping the head of the fibula. The first hand rotates the knee laterally, thus preventing posterior subluxation of the lateral condyle, while the second hand induces a valgus displacement. Under these conditions, the knee is extended while external rotation is checked and this combination of events is important for the test to be positive. As the knee is fully extended, the examiner's thumb pushes the fibula anteriorly. The test is positive when the *tibial plateau jerks anteriorly at the end of extension*.

The **drawer test of Noyes** (fig. 208) is also performed on a supine patient with *the knee at 20°–30° flexion and in neutral rotation*. The examiner's hands support the leg and the weight of the thigh causes *posterior subluxation of the lateral femoral condyle* (1) and *lateral rotation of the femur*. It is possible to reduce this subluxation by *pushing the superior end of the tibia posteriorly* (2), as one does when looking for the posterior drawer. The positive test also indicates rupture of the anterior cruciate.

Slocum's test (fig. 209) is performed on a supine patient half-turned to the opposite side. The examiner's hands lie on top of the limb under examination. The weight of the limb, when the knee is extended, automatically produces a combination of valgus displacement and medial rotation. There is no need to support the limb and this is useful when dealing with heavy patients. With his hands lying on either side of the joint space, the examiner flexes the knee while increasing the degree of valgus displacement. As in the McIntosh test, a sudden jerk appears at 30°–40° flexion and the converse is produced when the knee is extended, as in the Hughston test. A positive Slocum test indicates rupture of the anterior cruciate.

These five tests are very important for the demonstration of rupture of the anterior cruciate ligament but *they are unreliable under two conditions*:

in young girls with unduly lax joints, they can be falsely positive, and it is imperative to examine the other knee, which can also be unduly lax;

with a *severe tear of the posteromedial fibrotendinous sheet the lateral condyle is not checked* by the imposed valgus and the demonstration of the jerk can be very difficult.

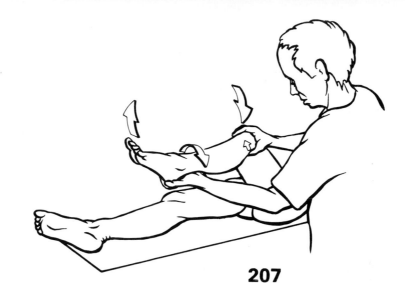

207

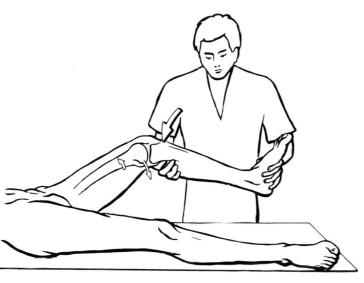

208

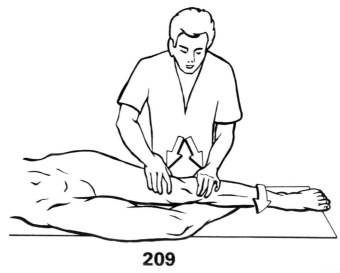

209

DYNAMIC TESTS OF THE KNEE: LATERAL ROTATION

Examination of the knee joint would be incomplete without dynamic tests associated with **lateral rotation**.

The **pivot shift reverse test** (fig. 210) is performed in the same way as the McIntosh test with lateral rotation replacing medial rotation. Starting from the position of flexion at 60°–90°, progressive extension, combined with pressure continuously applied to the lateral aspect of the knee, leads to the appearance of a jerk at less than 30° extension (fig. 211). This jerk is produced by a sudden shift of the lateral femoral condyle on to the posterior slope of the convex lateral tibial plateau.

When the laterally rotated knee is flexed (fig. 213), the lateral condyle, no longer held by the posterior cruciate during lateral rotation (LR), undergoes anterior subluxation (ASL) on the anterior slope of the convex tibial plateau (arrow 1). With further extension (fig. 212), the tensor fasciae latae (TFL) moves anterior to the point of contact between the condyle and the tibial plateau. As a result, the lateral condyle is pulled back posteriorly (fig. 213) into its normal position (shaded) and it abruptly crosses the ridge of the convex tibial plateau to land on its posterior slope (arrow 2). The sudden jerk can be perceived by the patient when the knee becomes unstable and by the observer during the test. It is caused by the *sudden reduction of the anterior subluxation of the lateral condyle*, secondary to **rupture of the posterior cruciate**.

The **combined lateral rotation-valgus-flexion test** (fig. 214) is performed in the same way but the *starting position is in full extension*. The jerk, obtained at 30° flexion (fig. 213), is caused by anterior subluxation (ASL) of the lateral condyle, which suddenly jumps from its normal position (arrow 2) on the posterior slope of the convex tibial plateau to an abnormal position (arrow 1) on the anterior slope. This can only occur after **rupture of the posterior cruciate**.

Three further tests allow the diagnosis of a *tear of the posterolateral sheet and of the lateral collateral ligament with an intact posterior cruciate*:

The **posterolateral drawer test of Hughston**: the feet are placed flat on the examining surface with the hips flexed at 45° and the knees at 90°. By sitting on the foot, the examiner is able to prevent knee rotation successively in the neutral position, in lateral rotation at 15° and in medial rotation at 15°. Holding the upper end of the tibia in both hands he can look for a posterior drawer in these three positions. The test is positive when there is *posterolateral subluxation of the lateral tibial plateau while the medial plateau stays put*. This produces a *true rotational drawer*, which decreases towards the neutral position and disappears with medial rotation as the intact posterior cruciate is stretched.

The **lateral hypermobility test of Bousquet** is done with *the knee flexed at 60°*. When pressure is applied to the superior end of the tibia in a attempt to displace it inferiorly and posteriorly with respect to the condyles, a posterior jerk is felt while the foot is being laterally rotated. This is an example of a *true lateral rotational drawer*.

The **recurvatum-lateral rotation test** can be performed in two ways while ensuring good relaxation of the quadriceps:

in *extension*: the lower limbs, held by the forefoot, are raised in extension and the abnormal limb displays a genu recurvatum and lateral rotation, produced by lateral displacement of the anterior tibial tuberosity. Posterolateral subluxation of the lateral tibial plateau produces genu varum;

in *flexion*: while the hand supports the foot and extends the knee, the other hand, holding the knee, can feel the posterolateral subluxation of the tibia, manifested as genu recurvatum, genu varum and lateral displacement of the anterior tibial tuberosity.

All these tests can be difficult to perform on a tense patient, but are easily performed **under general anaesthesia**.

134

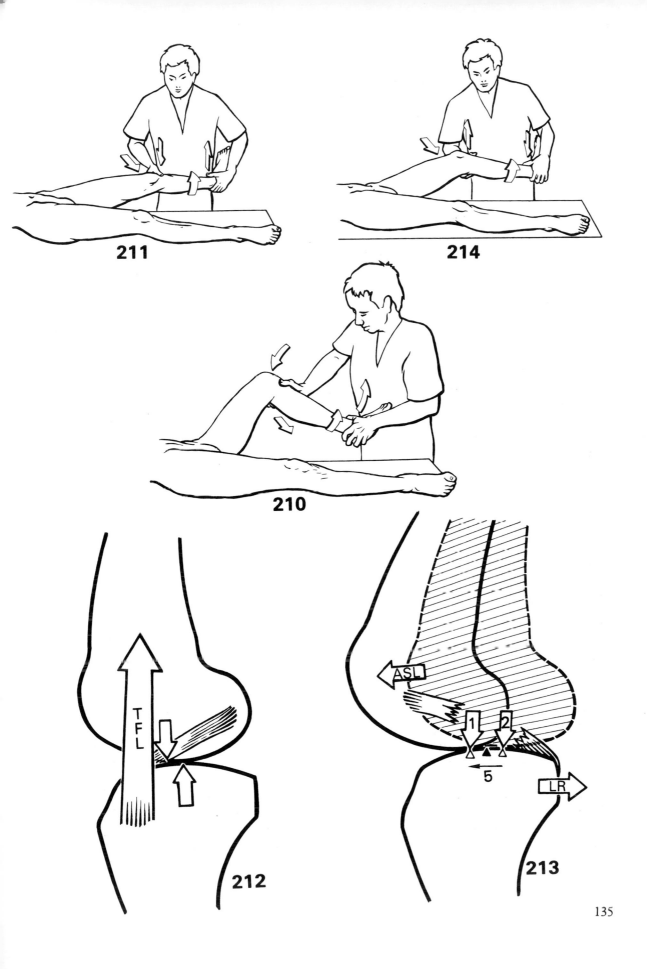

211

214

210

212

213

135

THE EXTENSOR MUSCLES OF THE KNEE

The **quadriceps femoris** is **the extensor muscle of the knee**. It is a *powerful muscle*: its active cross-sectional area is 148 cm^2 and, as *it shortens by a distance of* 8 cm., it develops a force equivalent to 42 kg. weight. It is *three times stronger* than the flexors, as can be expected from the fact that it counteracts the effect of gravity. We have already seen, however, that when the knee is hyperextended the quadriceps is not required for maintenance of the erect position (p. 110) but, as soon as flexion is initiated, the quadriceps is strongly thrown into action so as to prevent a fall resulting from knee flexion.

The quadriceps (fig. 215), as indicated by its name, consists of *four muscle bellies*, which are inserted by a common tendon into the anterior tibial tuberosity:

— three monoarticular muscles: the **vastus intermedius** (1), the **vastus lateralis** (2) and **the vastus medialis** (3);

— a biarticular muscle: the **rectus femoris** (4), whose very special functions will be studied on the next page.

These three monoarticular muscles are exclusively extensors of the knee, but they also exert a component of force sideways. It is worth noting that the medialis is more powerful and extends more distally than the lateralis and its relative predominance is meant to check lateral dislocation of the patella. The normally balanced contraction of these vasti produces *a resultant upward force along the long axis of the thigh* but, if there is imbalance of these muscles, e.g. if the vastus lateralis predominates over a deficient medialis, the patella 'escapes' laterally. This is one of the mechanisms responsible for *recurrent dislocation of the patella*, which always occurs laterally. Conversely, it is possible to correct this lesion by selectively strengthening the vastus medialis.

The patella is a **a sesamoid bone** embedded in the extensor tendon of the knee; its function is to increase the efficiency of the quadriceps *by shifting anteriorly the line of action of its muscular pull*. This is readily demonstrated by studying **the diagram of forces with and without the patella**.

The force Q of the quadriceps, acting on the patella (fig. 216), can be resolved into two vectors: a force Q1, acting towards the axis of flexion and extension and tending to keep the patella pressed against the femur, and a force Q2 acting along the line of the ligamentum patellae. This force Q2, acting on the tibial tuberosity, can also be resolved into *two vectors perpendicular to each other*: a force Q3, acting towards the axis of flexion and extension and keeping the tibia and femur together, and a tangential force Q4 which is *the component effective in extension*, i.e. it moves the tibia anteriorly underneath the femur.

Let us assume that the patella has been removed—i.e. after a patellectomy—and let us proceed as before (fig. 217). The force Q (assuming this one to be equal to the other Q) acts tangentially to the patellar surface of the femur and directly on the tibial tuberosity. It can therefore be resolved into two vectors: Q5, which keeps the tibia pressed against the femur, and Q6, the component effective for extension. Note that the tangential component of Q6 is clearly reduced whereas the centripetal component Q5 is relatively enhanced.

If we now compare the effective forces in these two situations (fig. 218), it is clear that Q4 is 50 per cent greater than Q6: thus *the patella, by raising the quadriceps tendon as on a trestle, increases its efficiency*. It is also evident that, in the absence of the patella, the force of coaptation Q5 is increased but this favourable effect is offset by the *reduction in the range of flexion* secondary to shortening of the extensor tendon and also *by the increased susceptibility to injury*. The patella is thus a very useful mechanical device and this explains the rarity and bad reputation of patellectomies.

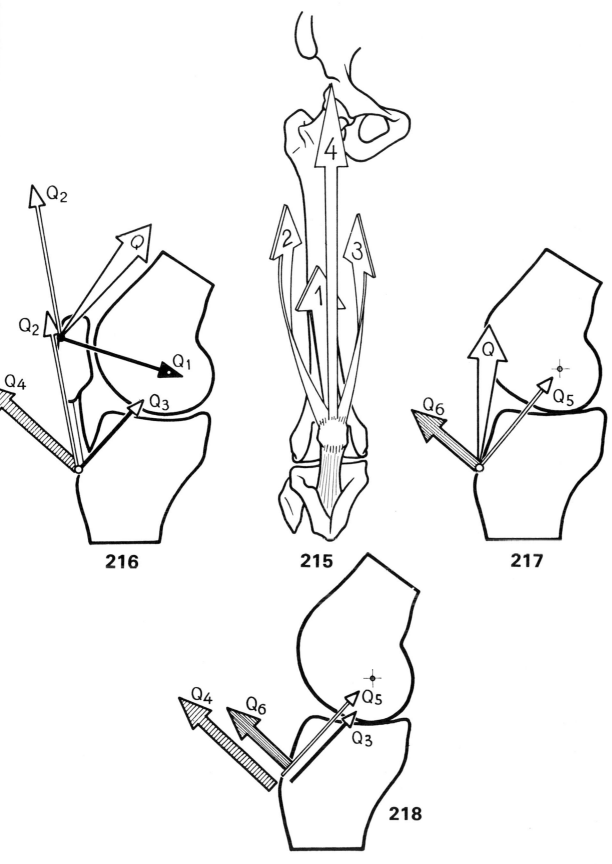

216

215

217

218

THE PHYSIOLOGICAL ACTIONS OF THE RECTUS FEMORIS

The rectus provides only *one-fifth* of the total force of the quadriceps and it cannot by itself produce full extension. But its biarticular nature gives it special significance.

As it runs anteriorly to the axis of flexion and extension of the hip and knee, it is at once a *flexor of the hip* and an *extensor of the knee* (fig. 220), but its efficiency as a knee extensor depends on the position of the hip and conversely its action as a hip flexor depends on the position of the knee. This is due to the fact (fig. 219) that the distance between the anterosuperior iliac spine (a) and the superior end of the patellar surface of the femur is shorter when the hip is flexed (ac) than when it is straight (ab). The difference (e) produces a *relative lengthening* of the muscle when the hip is flexed and the knee bends under the weight of the leg (II). Under these conditions, the vasti are more efficient in extending the knee (III) than the rectus, which is already slackened by hip flexion.

On the other hand, if the hip is extended (IV) from the reference position (I), the distance between the origin and insertion of the rectus (ad) increases by f and this stretches the rectus (i.e. relative shortening) and enhances its efficiency. This also occurs during running or walking when the posterior limb is lifted off the ground (fig. 223): the glutei extend the hip while the knee and ankle are flexed. The quadriceps then works at its best advantage because of the increased efficiency of the rectus. *The gluteus maximus is therefore an antagonist-synergist of the rectus femoris*, i.e. an antagonist at the hip and synergist at the knee.

When one limb moves forward off the ground (fig. 222), the pelvis being supported temporarily on the other hip, the rectus contracts to produce at once flexion of the hip and extension of the knee. Therefore the rectus, as a biarticular muscle, is useful in both phases of walking, i.e. when the posterior limb provides the propulsive thrust and when the anterior limb is moved forwards.

When one gets up from the crawling position, the rectus femoris plays an important role, since it is the only muscle of the quadriceps to maintain its efficiency throughout the movement. In effect, with the knee extended, the hip is also extended by the gluteus maximus, which *retightens the rectus at its origin*, thus ensuring constant length of the muscle early in contraction. Once more, we observe how the force generated by a powerful muscle at the root of the limb (the gluteus maximus) is allowed to act on a distal joint (the knee) via a biarticular muscle (the rectus femoris).

Conversely knee flexion produced by the hamstrings promotes hip flexion through the action of the rectus, which is useful during jumping with flexed knees (fig. 221). The recti thus contribute efficiently to hip flexion. This is yet another example of antagonism-synergism between the hamstrings, which flex the knee and extend the hip, and the rectus femoris, which flexes the hip and extends the knee.

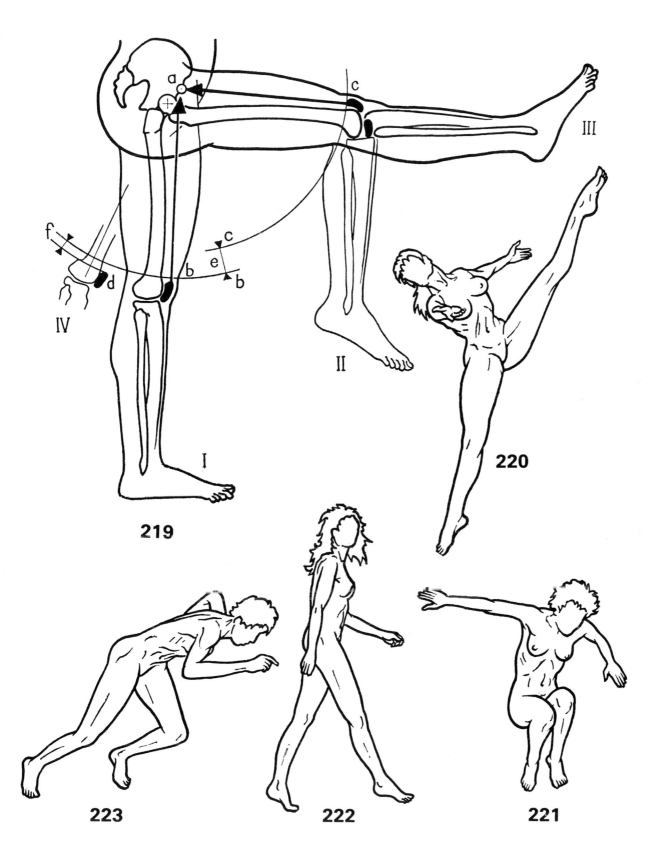

III

a

c

f

c

e

b

b

d

IV

II

220

I

219

223

222

221

THE FLEXOR MUSCLES OF THE KNEE

These are lodged in the **posterior compartment of the thigh** (fig. 224); they are the *hamstring muscles*—biceps femoris (1), semitendinosus (2), semimembranosus (3); the *three muscles inserted the medial aspect of the tibia*—the gracilis (4), sartorius (5) and semitendinosus (also part of the hamstrings); and the *popliteus*. The gastrocnemius (6 and 7) is practically useless as a knee flexor but is a powerful extensor of the ankle (p. 206).

The **gastroscnemius** is nevertheless a powerful stabiliser of the knee. With its insertion superior to the condyles, it contracts in the active phase of walking, i.e. when knee and ankle are extended simultaneously, and thus forces the condyles anteriorly. It is thus an *antagonist-synergist of the quadriceps*.

All these muscles are biarticular with two exceptions: the short head of the biceps and the popliteus which are monoarticular (p. 142). These biarticular flexors therefore also extend the hip simultaneously and their action on the knee depends on the position of the hip.

The **sartorius** (5) is a flexor, abductor and lateral rotator of the hip and at the same time a flexor of the knee.

The **gracilis** (4) is primarily an adductor and an accessory flexor of the hip; it also flexes the knee and participates in medial rotation of the knee.

The **hamstrings** are at once extensors of the hip (p. 42) and flexors of the knee and their action on the knee depends on the position of the hip (fig. 225). When the hip is flexed, the distance ab between the origins and insertions of these muscles increases progressively since the centre of the hip O, around which the femur turns, does not coincide with the point a around which the hamstrings turn. Thus the more the hip is flexed the greater the degree of relative shortening of these muscles and the more *stretched* they become. When the hip is flexed at 40° (II), the relative shortening of the muscles can be partly made up for by *passive* flexion of the knee (ab = ab'). However when hip flexion reaches 90° (III), the relative shortening cannot be wholly compensated even by a 90° flexion of the knee (f= 'residual' shortening). As hip flexion exceeds 90° (IV), it becomes very difficult to keep the knee in full extension (fig. 226): the amount of relative shortening (g) is just about absorbed by the **elasticity of the hamstrings**, which decreases remarkably with lack of exercise. **When the hamstrings are stretched by hip flexion their efficiency as knee flexors increases**: thus, during climbing (fig. 227) when one lower limb moves forward, flexion of the hip increases the efficiency of the knee flexors. Conversely, knee extension promotes the flexor action of these muscles on the hip: this occurs as one tries to straighten the trunk when it is bent forward (fig. 226) and when, during climbing, the posterior limb moves in front of the other limb.

If the hip is maximally extended (fig. 225, portion V) the hamstrings show a *relative lengthening* (3) and so they lose some of their efficiency (fig. 13) as knee flexors.

These observations stress the *usefulness of the monoarticular muscles* (popliteus and short head of biceps), which have the same efficiency whatever the position of the hip.

The total force produced by the flexors is equivalent to 15 kg. weight, i.e. about a third of that produced by the quadriceps.

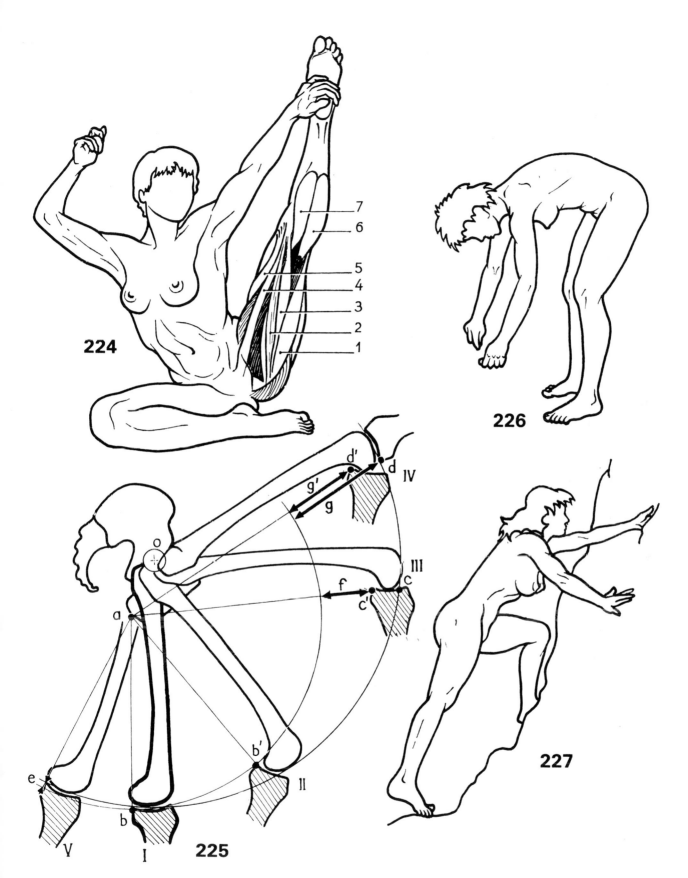

224

7
6
5
4
3
2
1

226

225

o

d′
g′
g
d IV

III
f
c
c′

a

b′

e

b
II

V
I

227

141

THE ROTATOR MUSCLES OF THE KNEE

The flexors are also at the same time **rotators** of the knee and they fall into two groups depending on their locus of insertion into the leg bones (fig. 228):

Those attached *lateral* (A) to the vertical axis XX' of rotation of the knee are **lateral rotators** (fig. 231), i.e. *biceps* (1) and *tensor fasciae latae* (2). When these muscles pull the lateral aspect of the tibial plateau posteriorly (fig. 239) they cause it to rotate so that the tips of the toes face more *laterally*. The tensor fasciae latae is only a flexor and lateral rotator when the knee is flexed; when it is fully extended the muscle loses its rotator action and becomes an extensor, i.e. it helps to 'lock' the knee in extension. The *short head of biceps* (fig. 232, I') is the only *monoarticular* lateral rotator and so the position of the hip has no effect on its function.

Those attached *medial* (B) to the vertical axis XX' of rotation of the knee are the *medial rotators* (fig. 231), i.e. the *sartorius* (3), *semitendinosus* (4), *semimembranosus* (5), *gracilis* (6) and *popliteus* (figs. 232, 7). When they pull posteriorly the medial aspect of the tibial plateau (fig. 230) they also cause it to rotate so that the tips of the toes now look *medially*. They act as *brakes on lateral rotation* taking place at the flexed knee and thus protect the capsule and ligaments when they are violently called into action during a violent turn to the side opposite the supporting limb.

The **popliteus** (fig. 234. seen from behind) is the only exception to this general mode of muscle distribution. Arising by tendon from the popliteal groove on the lateral surface of the lateral femoral condyle, it soon enters the *articular capsule*—still outside the synovium—to run between the lateral collateral ligament and the lateral meniscus (fig. 232). It sends a *fibrous expansion to the posterior edge of the lateral meniscus* and then emerges from the capsule under cover of the cruciate ligament (fig. 147) before reaching its insertion into the posterior aspect of the superior end of the tibia (the soleal line). Its action is easily understood from figure 233, which shows *the tibial plateau seen from above*. The popliteus (black arrow) pulls the posterior part of the tibial plateau laterally.

Although it lies posterior to the knee, the *popliteus is an extensor*. During flexion, its insertion shifts superiorly and anteriorly (fig. 232) and pulls on the muscle, thus *increasing its power as a medial rotator*. Conversely, when the knee is flexed or, even better, when the knee is laterally rotated, contraction of the popliteus pulls its insertion inferiorly and posteriorly, causing the lateral condyle to slide as it does during extension. Thus the popliteus is at once an extensor and a medial rotator of the knee.

The combined power of the medial rotators (2 kg. weight) is only a little greater than that of the lateral rotators (1·8 kg. weight).

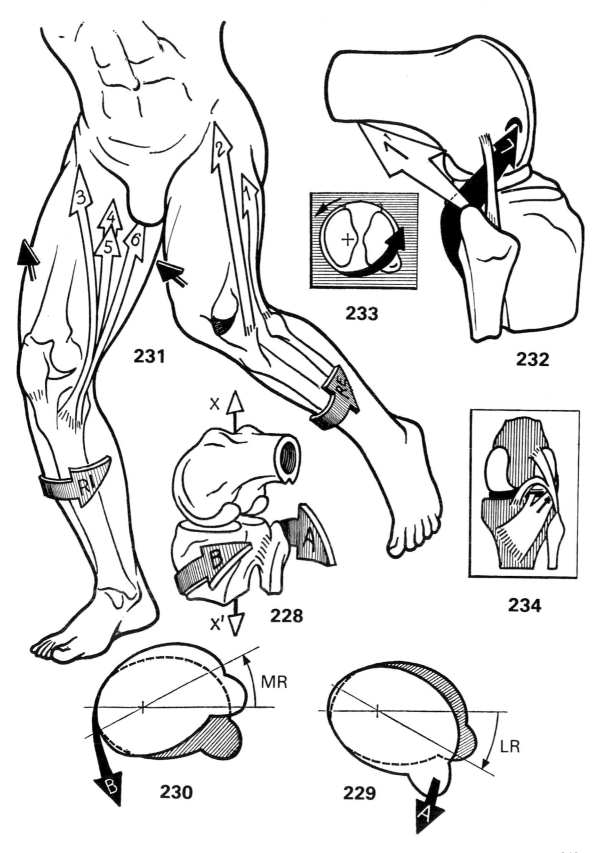

231

232

233

234

228

230

229

THE DYNAMIC EQUILIBRIUM OF THE KNEE

At the end of this chapter, it appears that the stability of this loosely-interlocked joint is a *miracle*. For this reason, we would like to provide a comprehensive diagram (fig. 245) that correlates the major clinical tests with the anatomical structures involved. The choice and the interpretation of these tests, based on recent publications, are debatable but this classification is offered as purely provisional.

1) the **direct anterior drawer test (neutral rotation)** can be weakly positive in normal subjects and comparison with the presumably normal side is essential. When it is obviously positive (+), it indicates *rupture of the anterior cruciate*. When it is strongly positive, it indicates combined *rupture of the medial collateral* and anterior cruciate ligaments. Beware of the false positive produced by spontaneous reduction of a posterior subluxation due to rupture of the posterior cruciate!

2) the **anterior drawer test (15° medial rotation)**, when positive, is a sure sign of *rupture of the anterior cruciate*, which may be coupled with *tearing of the posterolateral fibrotendinous sheet*.

3) the **anterior drawer test (30° medial rotation)**, when positive, indicates *combined rupture of both cruciate ligaments* and, if a jerk is present, there is also *tearing of the insertion of the posterior horn of the lateral meniscus*.

4) The **lateral jerk test (valgus-medial rotation-flexion)** or the lateral pivot shift test of McIntosh and the jerk test of Hughston, when positive, are diagnostic of *rupture of the anterior cruciate*.

5) The **anterior drawer test (external rotation)**, when moderately positive (+), indicates a tear of the posterolateral sheet and, if associated with a jerk, it implies *concurrent tearing of the insertion of the posterior horn of the medial meniscus*.

6) The **direct posterior drawer test (neutral rotation)**, when positive, indicates *rupture of the posterior cruciate*.

7) The **lateral jerk test (valgus-lateral rotation-extension/flexion)** or pivot shift reverse test, when positive, indicates *rupture of the posterior cruciate*.

8) The **posterior drawer test (lateral rotation)**, when positive, indicates a *tear of the posterolateral sheet* with or without *rupture of the posterior cruciate*.

9) The **posterior drawer test (medial rotation)**, when positive, is specific for *combined rupture of the posterior cruciate and of the posteromedial sheet*.

10) **Transverse lateral displacement in extension**, causing a slight degree of valgus (+), indicates *rupture of the medial collateral ligament*. When the valgus is moderate (++), there is an *associated fracture of the shell of the medial condyle*. When the valgus is severe (+++), there is also *rupture of the anterior cruciate*.

11) **Lateral displacement in weak flexion (10°–30°)** indicates *combined rupture of the medial collateral ligament, the shell of the medial condyle and of the posteromedial sheet as well as tearing of the posterior horn of the lateral meniscus*.

12) **Medial displacement in extension**, when the degree of associated varus is moderate (+), indicates *rupture of the lateral collateral ligament* with or without concurrent *rupture of the tensor fasciae latae*. When the varus is severe (++), there is an *associated rupture of the shell of the lateral condyle and of the posterolateral sheet*.

13) **Medial displacement in weak flexion (10°–30°)** indicates the same lesions *without rupture of the tensor fasciae latae*.

14) **The recurvatum-lateral rotation-valgus test**, when positive, indicates *combined rupture of the lateral collateral ligament and of the posterolateral sheet*.

To understand the mechanics of the knee, one must visualise the knee in terms of a **dynamic equilibrium** and, above all, one must give up the concept of bilateral equilibrium, represented by the two plates of a balance. Rather, *windsurfing* provides a closer analogy, with **three components in equilibrium**:

the sea, supporting the surfing board, corresponds to the *articular surfaces*.

the wind hitting the sail provides the motor-power and is analogous to the *muscles*.

the surfer, who guides the board by his constant reactions to sea and wind, corresponds to the *ligaments*.

Thus, at all times, the movements of the knee are determined by mutual and balanced interactions among these three factors, i.e. articular surfaces, muscles and ligaments — an example of **trilateral dynamic equilibrium**.

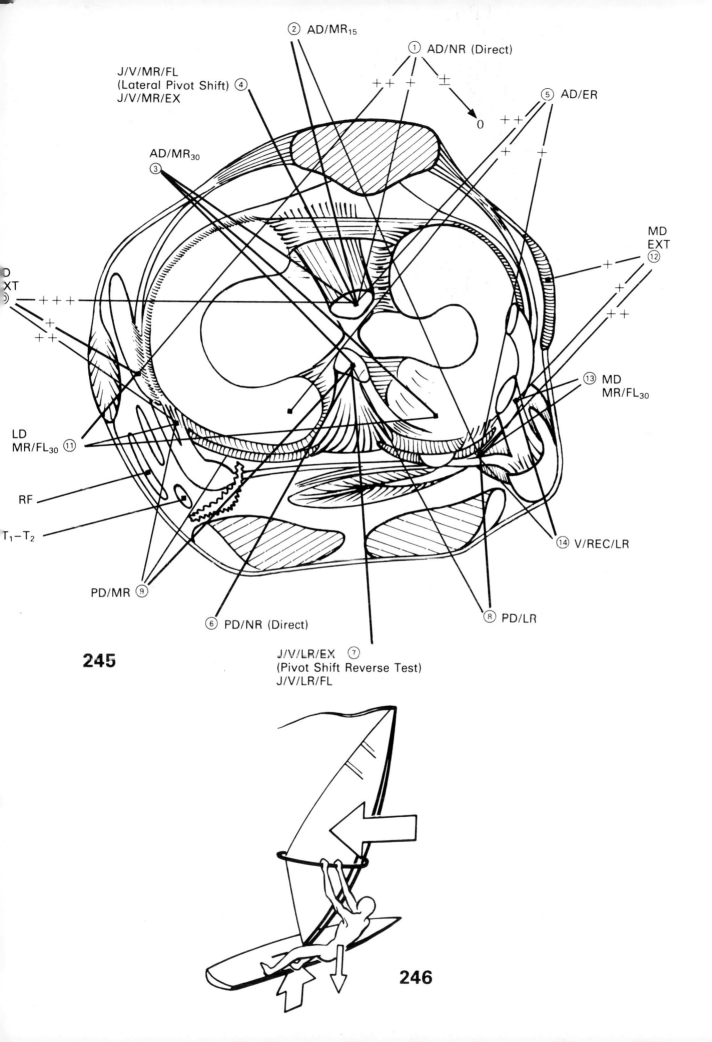

② AD/MR₁₅

① AD/NR (Direct)

J/V/MR/FL
(Lateral Pivot Shift) ④
J/V/MR/EX

⑤ AD/ER

AD/MR₃₀
③

MD
EXT
⑫

D
XT
⑩
+ + +
+
+ +

⑬ MD
MR/FL₃₀

LD
MR/FL₃₀ ⑪

RF

T₁–T₂

⑭ V/REC/LR

PD/MR ⑨

⑥ PD/NR (Direct)

⑧ PD/LR

245

J/V/LR/EX ⑦
(Pivot Shift Reverse Test)
J/V/LR/FL

246

The Ankle

The ankle or the tibiotarsal joint is the distal joint of the lower limb. It is a **hinge joint** and has therefore only *one degree of freedom*. It controls the movements of the leg relative to the foot, which occur in a *sagittal plane*. These movements are essential for walking on flat or rough ground.

It is a *tightly interlocled joint* exposed to extreme mechanical conditions during single limb support. It is then subjected to the entire body weight and to the force generated by the dissipation of kinetic energy when the foot rapidly makes contact with the ground during walking, running or jumping. It is thus easy to imagine the problems involved in the production of reliable longterm total prostheses for this joint.

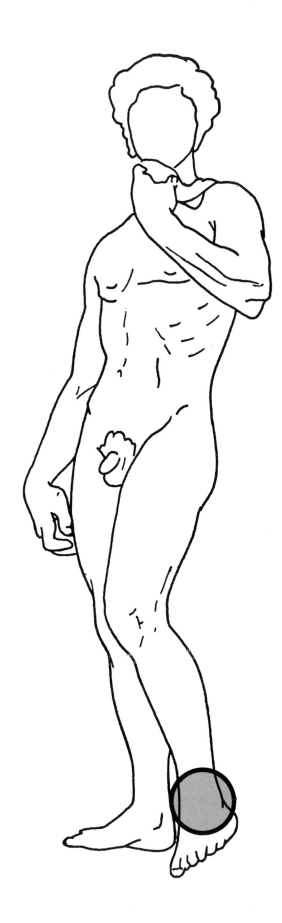

149

THE ARTICULAR COMPLEX OF THE FOOT

In fact, the ankle is only the most important of the joints of the posterior half of the foot. This series of joints, assisted by axial rotation of the knee, is in practice equivalent to a single joint with three degrees of freedom; it allows the foot to take up any position in space and to adapt to any irregularities of the ground. A certain similarity to the upper limb is evident: the joints of the wrist, assisted by pronation and supination, allow the hand to assume any position in space but the mobility of the hand is much greater than that of the foot.

The **three main axes** of this joint complex (fig. 1) intersect roughly in the posterior half of the foot. When the foot lies in the position of reference, the three axes are perpendicular one to another. In the diagram, extension of the ankle changes the direction of the Z axis.

The **transverse axis XX′** passes through the two malleoli and corresponds to the axis of the ankle proper. It lies almost wholly in the frontal plane and controls *the movements of flexion and extension* of the foot (p. 152), which occur in a sagittal plane.

The **long axis of the leg Y** is vertical and controls the *movements of adduction and abduction* of the foot, which take place in a transverse plane. As shown previously (p. 72), these are only possible because of axial rotation of the flexed knee. A smaller proportion of these movements of adduction and abduction depends on the joints of the posterior part of the foot but then they are always associated with movements around the third axis.

The **long axis of the foot Z** is horizontal and lies in a sagittal plane. It controls the movements of the sole of the foot and allows it to face inferiorly, laterally or medially. By analogy with the upper limb these movements can be called *pronation* and *supination* respectively.

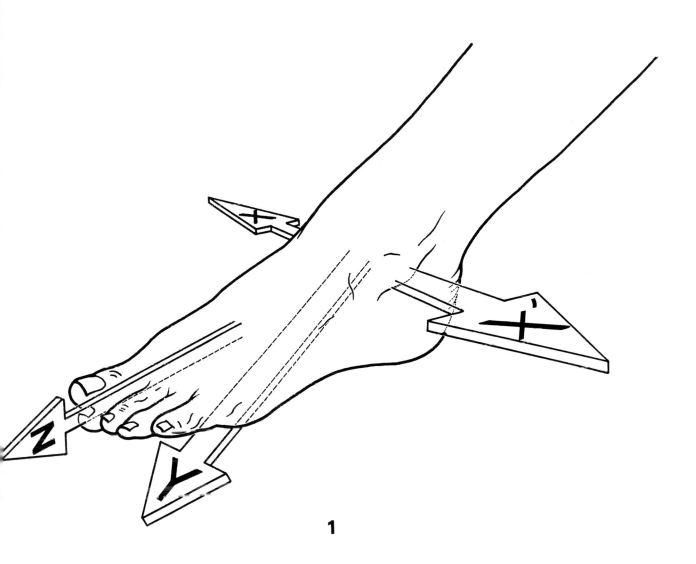

1

151

FLEXION AND EXTENSION

The **position of reference** (fig. 2) is achieved when the sole of the foot is perpendicular to the axis of the leg (A). From this position, **flexion of the ankle** (B) is the movement which approximates the dorsum of the foot and the anterior surface of the leg; it is also called dorsiflexion.

Conversely, **extension of the ankle** (C) is the movement of the dorsum of the foot away from the anterior surface of the leg so that the foot tends to fall into line with the leg. It is also called plantar flexion but this term is incorrect because flexion always corresponds to the movement of approximation of the segments of a limb and the trunk. In the diagram it is clear that the range of extension is distinctly greater than that of flexion. In measuring these angles, the centre of the ankle is not used as the reference point, as it is simpler to assess the angle between the sole of the foot and the axis of the leg (fig. 3).

When this angle is acute (b), **flexion** is present. Its range is from 20° to 30°. The striped zone indicates the range of individual variations, i.e. 10°.

When this angle is obtuse (c), **extension** is present. Its range is from 30° to 50°. The margin of individual variations, i.e. 20°, is greater than for flexion.

When these movements become extreme the ankle is not the only active joint: the tarsal joints contribute some range of movement, which is relatively small without being negligible. In extreme flexion (fig. 4), the tarsal joints contribute a few degrees (+) while the plantar arches are flattened. Conversely, during extreme extension (fig. 5) the increase in range (+) is provided by hollowing of the plantar arches.

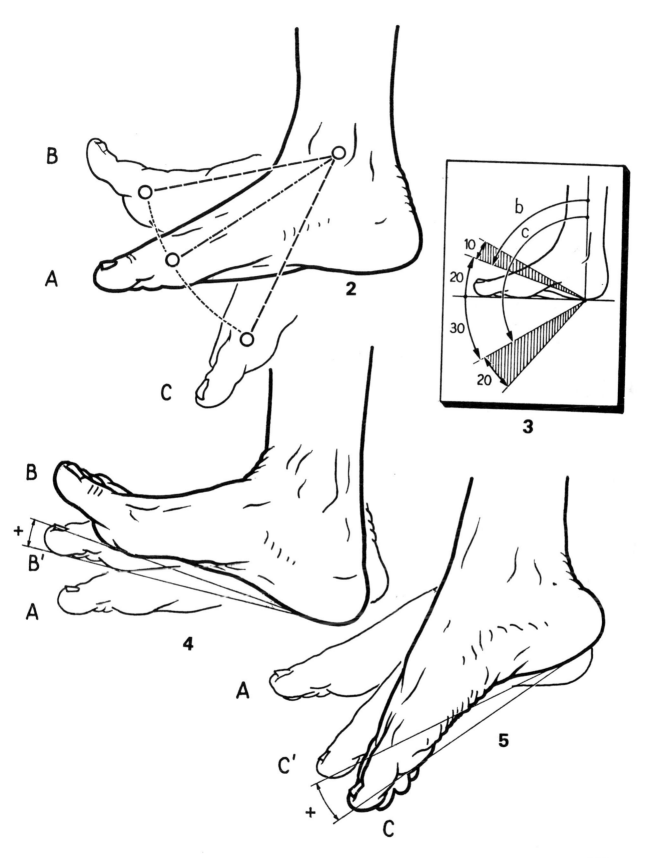

THE ARTICULAR SURFACES OF THE ANKLE

(The numbers have the same meaning in all the diagrams.)

If one compares the ankle to a **mechanical model** (fig. 6) it can be described as consisting of:

A lower structure (A), the talus, which bears on its superior aspect a roughly cylindrical surface with its long axis XX′ running transversely.

An upper structure (B), the distal end of the tibia and fibula, forming one structure (shown here as transparent): its lower surface contains a cylindrical cavity corresponding to the cylindrical upper surface of the talus.

The solid cylinder (A), encased within the cylindrical cavity of the upper structure (B), and kept in position by its two flanks, can perform movements of flexion (F) and of extension (E) *around a common axis XX′*.

In the **skeleton** (fig. 7: the ankle opened out and seen from in front and from inside; fig. 8: seen from behind and from inside) the solid cylinder corresponds to the **body of the talus** which has *three surfaces*: a superior or trochlear surface and a medial and a lateral surface.

The **superior or trochlear surface**, convex anteroposteriorly, is depressed centrally by a longitudinal groove—the *groove of the pulley* (1)—bounded by the medial (2) and lateral (3) lip of the pulley. As shown in figure 9 (seen from above), this groove does not strictly lie in a sagittal plane but runs obliquely anteriorly and laterally (arrow Z), along the long axis of the foot as the neck of talus faces anteriorly and medially (arrow T). Therefore the talus is twisted on itself. This diagram also shows that the trochlear surface is broader anteriorly (L) than posteriorly (*l*). This trochlear surface of the talus corresponds to a *reciprocally shaped* surface on the inferior aspect of the tibia (figs. 7 and 8) which is concave anteroposteriorly (fig. 12: sagittal section, viewed from the outside) and has a blunt sagittal ridge (4) to fit into the trochlear groove (fig. 11: frontal section, viewed from in front). One either side of this ridge, a medial (5) and a lateral (6) 'gutter' respectively receive the corresponding lips of the trochlear surface.

The **medial surface** (7) of the body of the talus (fig. 10) is nearly plane, except anteriorly, where it is inclined medially (fig. 7), and lies in a sagittal plane (fig. 9). It articulates with the facet (8) on the lateral surface of the medial malleous (9), which is lined by cartilage continuous with that lining the inferior surface of the tibia. The solid angle (10) lying between these two surfaces of the tibia receives the sharp border (11), which runs between the trochlear surface and the medial surface of the body of the talus.

The **lateral surface** (12) runs obliquely anteriorly and laterally (fig. 8) and is concave supero-inferiorly (fig. 11) as well as anteroposteriorly (fig. 9). It is in contact with the articular facet (13) of the medial surface (fig. 7) of the lateral malleolus (14). This facet is separated from the tibia by the line of the inferior tibiofibular joint (15), padded by a synovial fold (16) (p. 164), which articulates with the sharp border (17) running between the lateral and the trochlear surfaces of the body of the talus. This border is *bevelled* anteriorly (18) and posteriorly (19) (p. 162).

The medial and lateral surfaces of the body of the talus are hemmed in by the two malleoli which are basically different:

The lateral malleolus is bigger than the medial.

It extends farther distally (m, fig. 11).

It lies more posteriorly (fig. 9) so that it runs slightly obliquely (20°) laterally and posterior to the axis XX′.

The third malleolus (fig. 12) is occasionally used descriptively to mean the posterior edge of the lower end of the tibia (20), which sticks out more distally (p) than the anterior margin.

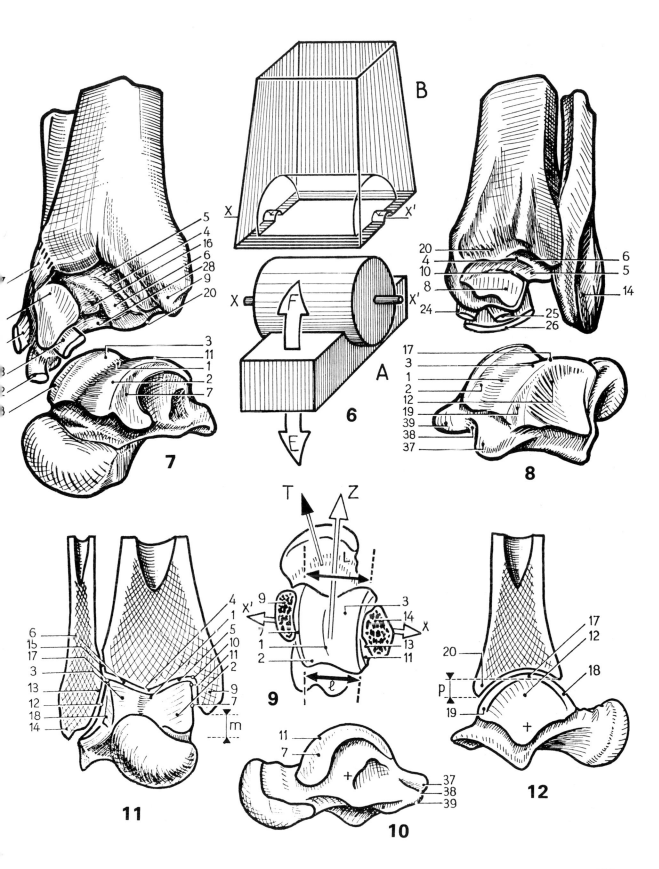

X

X'

B

X

X'

F

A

6

E

5
4
16
6
28
9
20

3
11
1
2
7

7

20
4
10
8
24

6
5
14
25
26

17
3
1
2
12
19
39
38
37

8

T
Z
L

9
7
1
2

X'
3
14
X
13
11

ℓ

9

6
15
17
3
13
12
18
14

4
1
5
10
11
2
9
7
m

11

11
7

+

37
38
39

10

20

P

19

17
12
18

+

12

155

THE LIGAMENTS OF THE ANKLE

(Diagrams are based on Rouvière; the numbers have the same meaning in all diagrams on this page and the preceding page.)

These ligaments consist of two main groups, i.e. the lateral and medial collateral ligaments, and two accessory groups, i.e. the anterior and posterior ligaments.

The **collateral ligaments** form on either side of the joint two powerful fan-like investments, which are attached above at their apices to the corresponding malleolus and which radiate out distally to be inserted into the two posterior tarsal bones.

The **lateral collateral ligament** (LCL) (fig. 13, seen from outside) is made up of three separate bands, two attached below to the talus and one to the calcaneus:

the **anterior talofibular ligament** (21), attached to the anterior margin of the fibular malleolus (14), runs obliquely inferiorly and anteriorly to be inserted into the talus between the lateral articular facet and the mouth of the sinus tarsi;

the **calcaneofibular ligament** (22), arising from the depression in front of the apex of the lateral malleolus, courses obliquely inferiorly and posteriorly to its insertion into the lateral surface of the calcaneus. The lateral talocalcanean ligament (32) runs along its inferior border;

the **posterior talofibular ligament** (23), arising from the medial surface of the lateral malleolus behind the articular facet, runs horizontally and inclines medially and slightly posteriorly to its insertion into the posterolateral tubercle of the talus (37). Because of its position and direction it is more easily seen from behind (fig. 14). It is prolonged by the posterior talocalcanean ligament (31).

From the lateral malleolus spring two other ligaments (figs. 14 and 15): the anterior (27) and posterior (28) inferior tibiofibular ligaments; their significance will emerge later.

The **medial collateral ligament** (MCL) (fig. 16: seen from inside), comprises two sets of fibres, superficial and deep.

The deep fibres consist of two talotibial bands:

the **anterior talotibial ligament** (25) runs obliquely inferiorly and anteriorly to be attached to the medial aspect of the neck of the calcaneus;

the **posterior talotibial ligament** (24) runs obliquely inferiorly and posteriorly to be inserted into a deep fossa (fig. 10) on the medial surface of the calcaneus; its most posterior fibres are attached to the posteromedial tubercle (39).

The superficial fibres, triangular in shape, and broad, constitute the **deltoid ligament** (26). In figure 15 (seen from the front) the deltoid ligament has been notched and retracted to demonstrate the deep posterior talofibular ligaments (25) and in figure 16 (seen from the inside) it is shown as a transparent structure. From its origin on the medial malleolus (36) it fans out and is inserted into a continuous line running from the tuberosity of the navicular bone (33), along the medial margin (34) of the plantar calcaneonavicular ligament (p. 178), to the sustentaculum tali of the calcaneus (35). Thus the deltoid ligament, like the lateral ligament, is not attached to the talus.

The **anterior** (fig. 15, seen from in front) and **posterior** (fig. 14, seen from behind) **ligaments** of the ankle are simply localised thickenings of the capsule. The *anterior* ligament (29) runs obliquely from the anterior margin of the lower end of the tibia to the upper surface of the anterior part of the neck of the talus (fig. 13). The *posterior* ligament (30) consists of fibres which spring from the tibia and the fibula and coverge to their insertion into the posteromedial tubercle of the talus (39). This tubercle, along with the posterolateral tubercle, forms the deep groove for the flexor hallucis longus (38); this groove is seen to proceed distally along the inferior surface of the sustentaculum tali.

156

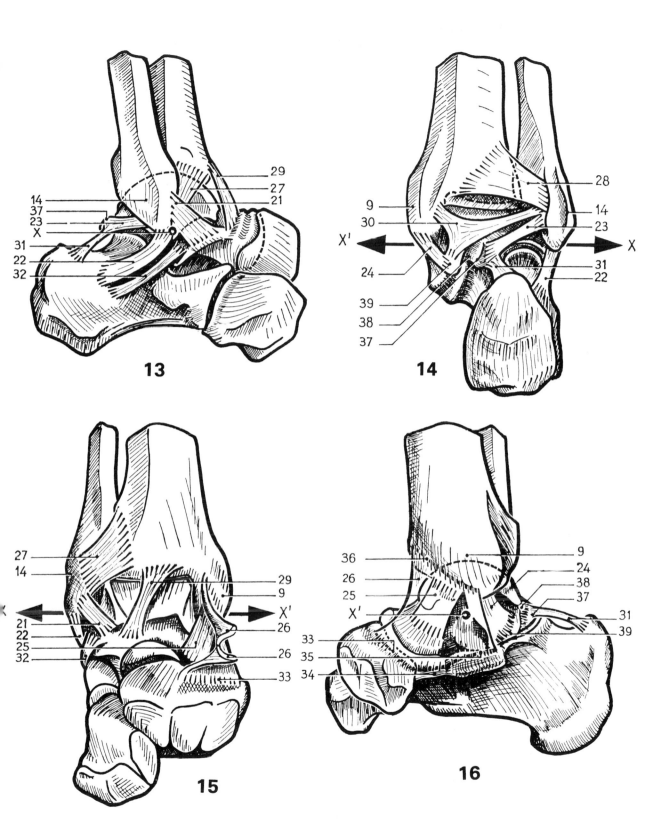

13

14

15

16

THE ANTEROPOSTERIOR STABILITY OF THE ANKLE AND THE FACTORS LIMITING FLEXION AND EXTENSION

The range of the movements of flexion and extension is first of all determined by the 'lengths' of the profiles of the articular surfaces (fig. 17). The tibial surface is equivalent to the arc of a circle subtending an angle of 70° at the centre and the trochlear surface of the talus to an arc subtending an angle of 140° to 150°, therefore by simple arithmetic the total range of flexion and extension can be deduced to be 70° to 80°. Since the 'arc length' of the trochlear surface is longer posteriorly than anteriorly it follows that extension has a greater range than flexion.

Flexion is checked (fig. 18) by the following factors:

bony factors: during extreme flexion the upper surface of the neck of the talus comes into contact (1) with the anterior margin of the tibial surface. If flexion continues, the neck of the talus can be fractured. The inferior part of the capsule is prevented from being nipped between the two bones by being pulled up (2) by the flexor muscles, whose sheaths are attached to the capsule;

capsular and ligamentous factors: the posterior part of the capsule is stretched (3) as well as the posterior fibres of the collateral ligaments (4);

one muscular factor: the resistance offered by the tonically active soleus and gastrocnemius muscles (5) usually limits flexion before the other two factors. Hence shortening of these muscles will check flexion prematurely and the ankle may be fixed permanently in a position of extension (talipes equinus); this can be corrected surgically by lengthening the Achilles tendon.

Extension is checked (fig. 19) by similar factors:

bony factors: the posterior tubercles of the talus, especially the posterolateral tubercle, strike (1) the posterior margin of the tibial surface. Occasionally the posterolateral tubercle is fractured during hyperextension but very often this tubercle is separate from the talus and is called the os trigonum. Once more the capsule avoids being nipped (2) by a mechanism similar to that operating during flexion;

capsular and ligamentous factors: the anterior part of the capsule is stretched (3) as well as the anterior fibres of the collateral ligaments (4);

a muscular factor: the resistance offered by the tonically active flexor muscles (5) is the first limiting factor. Hyperactivity of the flexors leads to a flexion of deformity of the ankle (talipes calcaneus).

The anteroposterior stability of the ankle and the coaptation of its articular surfaces (fig. 20) depend upon the effect of *gravity* (1), which keeps the talus pressed against the distal surface of the tibia while the *anterior* (2) and *posterior* (3) *margins* of the tibial surface form bony spurs which prevent the talar pulley from escaping anteriorly or posteriorly. The *collateral ligaments* (4) are passively responsible for the coaptation of the surfaces and are assisted by the muscles (not shown here), provided the joint is intact.

When flexion and extension exceed the normal range, one of the limiting factors must give way. Thus, during **hyperextension**, the joint may be dislocated posteriorly (fig. 21) with partial or complete disruption of the capsular ligaments or the posterior margin of the tibial surface (fig. 22) or third malleolus may be fractured with secondary posterior subluxation of the joint. This subluxation tends to recur even after proper surgical reduction, if the 'arc length' of the fractured margin exceeds one-third of the 'arc length' of the tibial surface; fixation by pinning becomes imperative. Likewise, during **hyperflexion**, the joint may be dislocated anteriorly (fig. 23) or there may be fracture of the anterior margin of the tibial surface (fig. 24).

When the lateral collateral ligament is sprained, the anterior band (fig. 25) is the first to be affected. It is simply pulled in a *minor sprain* and torn in a *severe sprain*. It is possible, clinically and better radiologically, to demonstrate a **drawer anterior** to the ligament. The talus escapes anteriorly and the circular surfaces of the tenon-like talus and of the mortise-like tibia are no longer concentric. When their centres of curvature are staggered by more than 4–5 mm., rupture of the anterior band of the lateral collateral ligament has occurred.

158

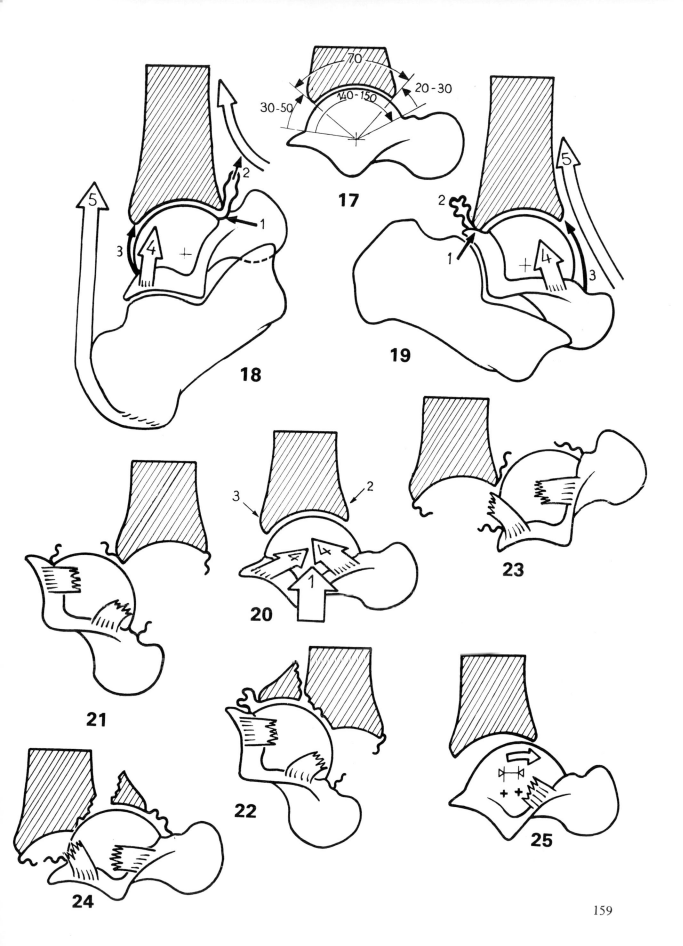

17

18

19

20

21

22

23

24

25

159

THE TRANSVERSE STABILITY OF THE ANKLE

Being a joint with a single degree of freedom, the ankle cannot, by virtue of its very structure, exhibit movements around its two other axes in space. This stability depends upon the **tight interlocking of its surfaces**: in fact it is analogous to a *tenon-and-mortise joint*, with the talar tenon being tightly fitted into the tibiofibular mortise (fig. 26). The two malleoli, as the two branches of a *pincer*, grip the talus on each side provided that the distance between the lateral (A) and medial (B) malleoli is unchanged. This condition is fulfilled only when the malleoli and the ligaments of the inferior tibiofibular joint (1) are intact. Furthermore the powerful lateral (2) and medial (3) collateral ligaments preclude any rolling movement of the talus about its long axis.

When a **violent movement of abduction** takes place, i.e. the foot is forcibly moved laterally, the lateral surface of the talus strikes against the lateral malleolus and the following consequences may ensue:

the 'malleolar pincer' is disrupted (fig. 27) as a result of rupture of ligaments of the inferior tibiofibular joint (1), this leads to widening of the tibiofibular mortise or **diastasis of the ankle**. Thus the talus is no longer held tightly and can move from side to side (rattling of the talus). It can also (fig. 28) rotate about its long axis (tilting of the talus) and this is made easier if the medial collateral ligament (MCL) is sprained (3) (in the diagram the ligament is shown stretched, i.e. a mild sprain). Finally, the talus can turn (fig. 33) round its vertical axis (arrow Abd) so that the posterior part of the trochlear surface of the talus fractures the *posterior margin* of the tibial surface (arrow 2);

if this movement of abduction continues (fig. 32) the medial collateral ligament (3) is torn: this is the *severe sprain* of the medial ligament associated with diastasis of the ankle;

or else the medial malleolus (B) snaps (fig. 30) at the same time as the lateral malleolus (A) snaps above the inferior tibiofibular joint (1). This represents one form of **Pott's fracture**. Occasionally the fibular fracture occurs much higher at the level of the neck: this is Maisonneuve's fracture (not shown here);

very often the inferior tibiofibular ligaments resist tearing (fig. 29), especially the anterior. Fracture of the medial malleolus (B) is then associated with fracture of the lateral malleolus *before or through the inferior tibiofibular joint*. This is another form of **Pott's fracture**. Occasionally the medial malleolus fails to snap (fig. 31) and the medial collateral ligament is ruptured (3). In these types of fracture a chip of bone is frequently broken off the 'third malleolus' (posterior margin of the tibia): this can be a separate fragment or it may form a single unit with the malleolar fragment.

In addition to these abduction dislocations and fractures, there are also **bimalleolar adduction fractures** (fig. 34). As the foot is adducted the talus (fig. 33) is made to rotate about its vertical axis (arrow Add) and its medial surface breaks off (arrow 3) the medial malleolus (B). The talus is also tilted at the same time and this leads to fracture of the lateral malleolus (A) at the level of the tibial articular surface.

Most of the time, however, this movement of adduction causes not a fracture but a **sprain of the lateral collateral ligament**. In most cases fortunately, this sprain is mild, with stretching rather than rupture of the ligament. On the other hand, in severe sprains the lateral collateral ligament is torn, leading to instability of the ankle. An **antero-posterior radiograph** taken in forced adduction (achieved, if necessary, under general anaesthesia) will show (fig. 35) **tilting of the talus**. The two articular surfaces of the joint are no longer parallel, but lie at an angle of over $10°-12°$ open laterally. Some ankles may be unusually lax and it is advisable to have a radiograph of the other presumably normal ankle for comparison.

It goes without saying that all these lesions of the 'malleolar pincer' require proper treatment if one is to restore the structural and functional integrity of the ankle joint.

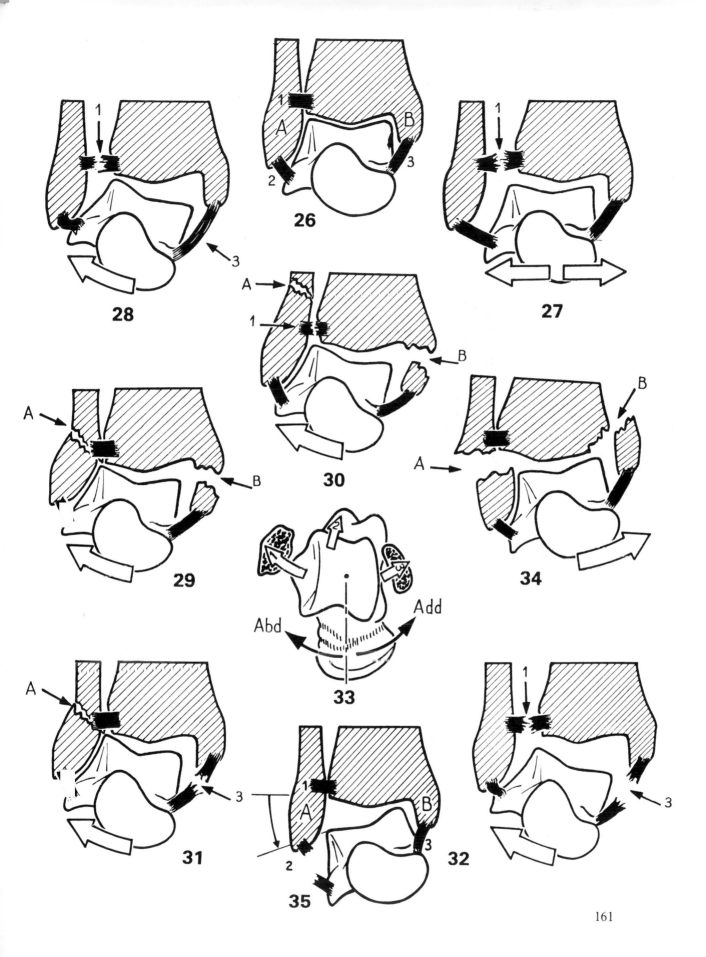

26

28

27

30

29

34

33

Abd Add

31

35

32

161

THE TIBIOFIBULAR JOINTS

The tibia articulates with the fibula at its two extremities, i.e. at the superior tibiofibular joint (figs. 36 to 38) and the inferior tibiofibular joint (figs. 39 to 41). It will be shown in the next page that these two joints are *mechanically linked to the ankle* and it is therefore logical to study these two joints in relation to the ankle.

The **superior tibiofibular joint** is clearly exposed (fig. 36) when the fibula is rotated after sectioning the anterior ligament (1) and the anterior expansion (2) of the biceps tendon (3). The joint then opens out around the hinge formed by its posterior ligament (4). It is a *plane joint* with oval articular surfaces which are plane or slightly convex. The tibial articular facet (5) lies on the posterolateral aspect of the rim of the tibial condyle; it faces obliquely posteriorly, inferiorly and laterally (arrow). The fibular facet (5) lies on the upper surface of the head of the fibula and it looks anteriorly, superiorly and medially. It is overhung by the styloid process of the fibula (7) which gives insertion to the tendon of the biceps femoris (3). The lateral collateral ligament of the knee joint (8) is attached between the biceps insertion and the fibular facet. Figure 37 (seen from behind) shows clearly how far posteriorly the fibular head lies; it also shows the anterior ligament of the joint (1), which is short and quadrilateral, and the thick tendinous expansion of the biceps (2) which runs to its insertion into the lateral condyle of the tibia. Figure 38 (seen from behind) illustrates the intimate relation of the popliteus (9) with the superior tibiofibular joint as it runs superficial to the posterior ligament (4).

The **inferior tibiofibular joint** (fig. 39: opened as before) contains no articular cartilage and is therefore a *syndesmosis*. The tibial facet (1) is the rough concave fibular notch of the tibia bounded by the two lips of the lateral border of the tibia. The fibular facet (2) is convex, plane or even concave and is continuous below with the cartilage-lined fibular articular facet (3) of the ankle which gives attachment to the posterior talofibular band (4) of the lateral collateral ligament. The *anterior ligament* of the inferior tibiofibular joint (5), thick and pearly, runs obliquely inferiorly and laterally (fig. 40, seen from in front). Its inferior border overlaps the tibiofibular mortise laterally and so during flexion of the ankle it 'nicks' the lateral ridge of the tochlear surface of the talus (double arrow). The *posterior ligament* (6), thicker and broader (fig. 41: seen from behind), runs a long way towards the medial malleolus; likewise it 'nicks' the posterior part of the lateral ridge of the trochlear surface of the talus during ankle extension.

In addition to the ligament of the joint, the two bones are joined by the **interosseous ligament** between the fibular notch of the tibia and the inner surface of the fibula (heavy dotted lines in figs. 36 and 39).

In the inferior tibiofibular joint the two bones are not in contact with each other: they are held apart by fibro-adipose tissue and this gap can be shown on radiographs properly centred on the ankle (fig. 42). Normally the shadow of the fibula (c) encroaches upon the anterior border (a) of the fibular notch of the tibia by 8 mm., which it is only 2 mm. away from the posterior border of the fibular notch (b). If the distance cb is greater than ac, then *diastasis of the ankle joint* is said to be present.

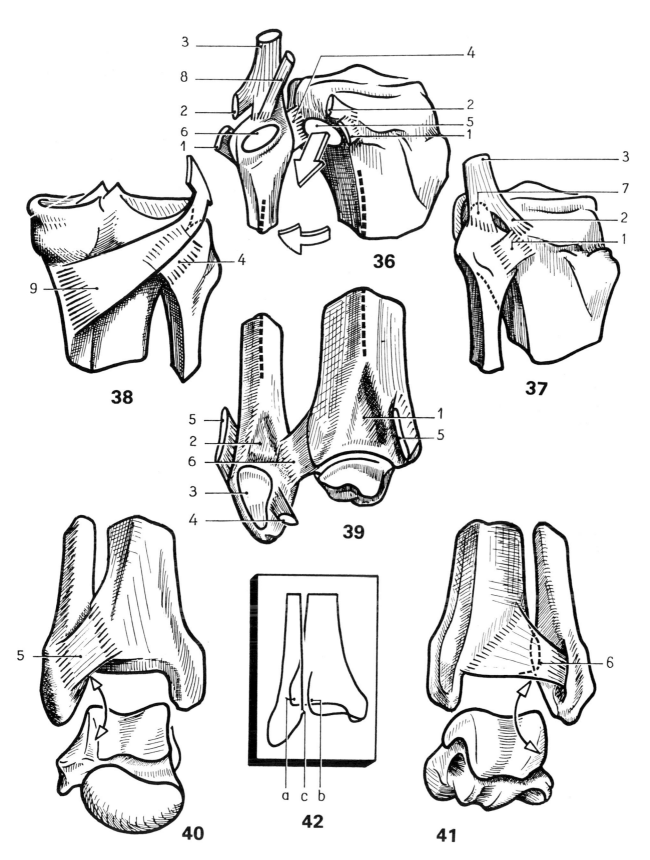

3
8
2
6
1

4
2
5
1

36

4

9

38

3
7
2
1

37

5
2
6
3
4

1
5

39

5

40

a c b

42

6

41

THE PHYSIOLOGICAL FUNCTIONS OF THE TIBIOFIBULAR JOINT

Flexion and extension of the ankle automatically call into action the two tibiofibular joints which are therefore **mechanically linked** to the ankle.

The **inferior tibiofibular joint** is the first to be recruited. Its mode of action has been well worked out by Pol le Coeur (1938) and depends essentially on the shape of the trochlear surface of the talus (fig. 43: seen from above). Its medial surface (M) lies in a sagittal plane while the lateral surface (L) lies in a plane which runs obliquely anteriorly and laterally. Therefore the width of the trochlear surface is smaller (posteriorly (aa') than anteriorly (bb')) by 5 mm. Hence, if the medial and lateral surfaces of the body of the talus are to be gripped tightly the **intermalleolar space must vary within certain limits**, i.e. being smallest during extension (fig. 44: seen from below) and greatest during flexion (fig. 45). On the cadaver, the ankle can be extended simply by pressing the malleoli firmly together.

In the anatomical model (figs. 44 and 45) it is also obvious that this movement of separation and approximation of the malleoli is associated with **axial rotation of the lateral malleolus**, while the posterior ligament of the tibiofibular joint (1) acts as a hinge. This rotation is easily demonstrated by the use of a pin which is driven horizontally through the lateral malleolus. When moving from the position of flexion (mm', fig. 45) to a position of extension (nn', fig. 44) the malleolus is medially rotated over 30°. At the same time the posterior ligament of the tibiofibular joint (2) is stretched, Note that this medial rotation of the malleolus is less marked in life but is nevertheless present. The synovial fringe (f) contained within the joint is displaced as follows: when the malleoli are approximated during extension (fig. 46) it is forced out distally (1); during flexion (fig. 47) it is pulled up (2).

Finally the fibula **moves vertically superiorly and inferiorly** (figs. 48 and 49: the fibula is represented by a ruler). Being attached to the tibia by the fibres of the interosseous membrane which run obliquely inferiorly and laterally (for clarity's sake only one fibre is shown), the fibula is lifted slightly as it moves away from the tibia (fig. 49) and is pulled down as it draws near to the tibia (fig. 48). To sum up the movements of the fibula:

During flexion of the ankle (fig. 50):

the lateral malleolus moves *away* from the medial malleolus (arrow 1).

at the same time it is slightly *pulled superiorly* (arrow 2) while the fibres of the tibiofibular and interosseous ligaments tend to become horizontal (xx');

finally, the fibula is *medially rotated* (arrow 3).

During extension of the ankle (fig. 51) the converse takes place:

the malleoli are approximated *actively* (arrow 1): contraction of the posterior tibialis with its fibres inserted into these two bones tightens the 'malleolar pincer' (fig. 52: section of the lower fragment of the right leg; the arrows show the contraction of the fibres of the posterior tibialis). Thus the body of the talus is well held in, whatever the degree of flexion or extension of the ankle;

the lateral malleolus is pulled *inferiorly* (arrow 2) while the ligaments tend to become vertical yy';

the malleolus is slightly *rotated medially* (arrow 3).

The **superior tibiofibular joint** is called into action as a result of movements of the lateral malleolus: during flexion of the ankle (fig. 50) the fibular facet slides superiorly and the joint interspace opens out to form an angle facing inferiorly (separation of the malleoli) and posteriorly (medial rotation of the fibula); during extension (fig. 51) the exact converse occurs.

These displacements are very small but they occur, and the best proof of their significance is to be found in the fact that during evolution the superior tibiofibular joint has not undergone ankylosis.

Thus by means of the tibiofibular joints, the ligaments and the tibialis posterior the 'malleolar pincers' can constantly adapt to the changes in width and curvature of the tenon-like talus and ensure the transverse stability of the ankle. It is mainly for the purpose of maintaining this adaptability that pinning operations have lost favour in the management of diastasis of the ankle.

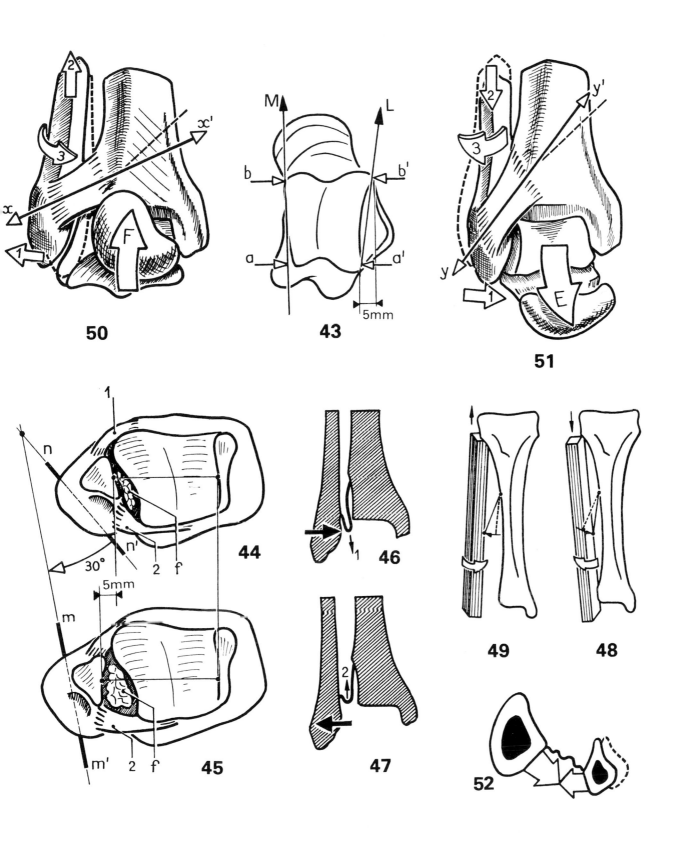

50

43

51

44

45

46

47

49

48

52

165

The Foot

The joints of the foot are many and complex and fall into two main groups: the intertarsal joints and the tarsometatarsal joints. The important joints are the following:

the talocalcanean or subtalar joint;

the midtarsal or transverse tarsal joint;

the tarsometatarsal joint;

the cubonavicular joint and the cuneonavicular joint.

These joints perform a *dual function*.

Firstly, they orientate the foot with respect to the other two axes in space (the ankle controls movements of the foot in the sagittal plane) so that the sole of the foot is correctly presented to the ground, whatever the position of the leg and the slope of the ground.

Secondly, they alter the shape and curvature of the arches of the foot so that the foot can adapt to the irregularities of the ground; they thus interpose a shock-absorber between the ground and the weight-bearing foot and impart greater elasticity and suppleness to the step.

These joints, therefore, play a vital part in the foot. On the other hand the metatarosphalangeal and interphalangeal joints are far less important than their counterparts in the hand.

One of these joints, however, is critical when a step is taken and it is the **metatarsophalangeal joint of the big toe**.

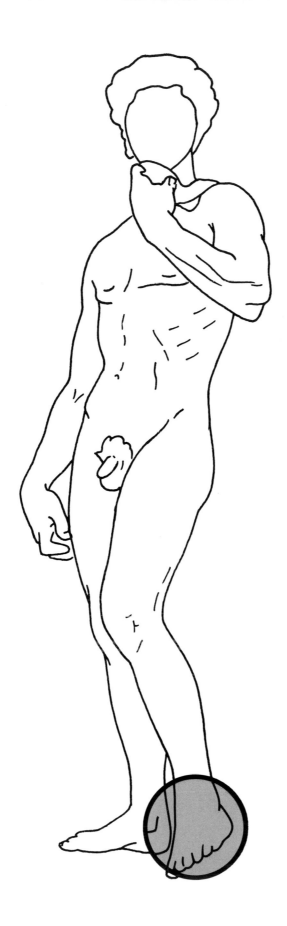

THE MOVEMENTS OF LONGITUDINAL ROTATION AND THE TRANSVERSE MOVEMENTS OF THE FOOT

In addition to movements of flexion and extension, which occur at the ankle, the foot can move about the vertical axis of the leg (axis Y, p. 150) and about its own horizontal and longitudinal axis (axis Z).

About the vertical axis Y occur movements of **adduction** and **abduction**:

adduction (fig. 2): when the tips of the toes move towards the plane of symmetry of the body and face inwards;

abduction (fig. 3): when the tips of the toes move away from the plane of symmetry and point outwards.

The total range of these movements, when they occur exclusively in the foot, is from 35° to 45° (Roud). However, these movements of the tips of the toes in the horizontal plane can also be achieved by lateral or medial rotation of the leg (knee flexed) or by rotation of the whole lower limb from the hip (knee extended). They have then a much greater range, attaining a maximum of 90° each way in ballerinas.

About the longitudinal axis Z the foot can turn so that the sole of the foot can face either:

medially (fig. 4): by analogy with the upper limb this is *supination*;

laterally (fig. 5): *pronation*.

The range of supination is 52° (Biesalski and Mayer, 1916) and is greater than that of pronation (25° to 30°).

These movements of adduction and abduction and rotation, as defined, do not in life occur *exclusively in the joints of the foot*. In fact, it will be shown later that movements in any one of the planes must needs be associated with movements in the other two planes. Thus adduction is necessarily accompanied (figs. 2 and 4) by supination and a slight measure of extension. These three component movements are characteristic of the position known as *inversion*. If the extension component is cancelled by flexion of the ankle the position of the foot is known as *talipes varus*. Finally if lateral rotation at the knee compensates for adduction of the foot, then the movement of *apparently pure supination* is produced.

Conversely (figs. 3 and 5), abduction is necessarily associated with pronation and flexion: this leads to *eversion*. If the flexion component is cancelled by extension of the ankle (in the diagrams it is overcompensated in extension) the position of *talipes valgus* is obtained. If in addition medial rotation of the knee makes up for abduction of the foot, then a movement of *apparently pure pronation* is achieved.

Thus, barring any compensatory movements occurring at joints outside the foot, adduction can never be associated with pronation and, vice versa, abduction can never be associated with supination. Therefore there are in the foot *forbidden combinations* of movement resulting from the very structure of its joints.

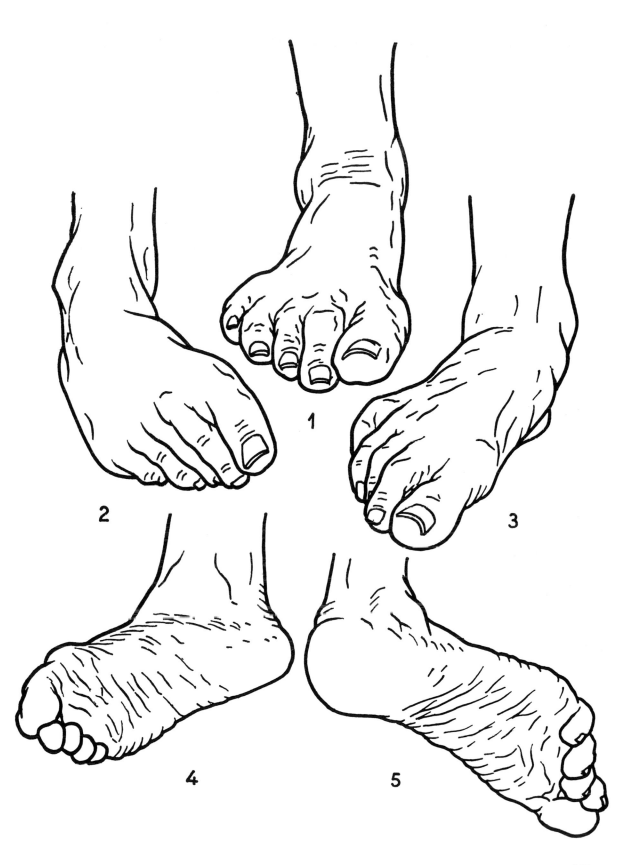

1

2   3

4   5

THE SUBTALAR (TALOCALCANEAN) JOINT: THE ARTICULAR SURFACES
(the numbers have the same meaning in all the diagrams)

The inferior surface of the talus articulates (A, fig. 6: the bones have been separated and the talus rotated around its hinge-like axis xx') with the superior surface of the calcaneus (B, fig. 6). This occurs at two separate articular facets, which constitute together **the subtalar joint**:

The posterior surface of the talus (a) is in contact with the broad (a') superior surface of the calcaneus (also known as the thalamus of Destot). These two surfaces are united by ligaments and a capsule, so that the joint is anatomically distinct.

The small surface (b) on the inferior surface of the neck and head of the talus rests on the anterior surface of the calcaneus (b'), which is obliquely set and is supported by the sustentaculum tali and the neck of the calcaneus. The joint, however, also includes the posterior surface of the navicular bone (d') which articulates with the head of the talus (d). This joint, properly the talocalcaneonavicular joint, is the most medial of the mid-tarsal joints.

Before studying the function of these joints, the shape of their articular surfaces must be understood.

These joints are of the **plane variety**:

The superior surface of the calcaneus (a') is roughly oval with its great axis running anterolaterally; it is convex about this great axis and plane or slightly concave about the other axis (fig. 7: seen from outside; fig. 8: seen from inside). Therefore it can be viewed as analogous to a segment of a cylinder (f) with its axis running obliquely postero-anteriorly, lateromedially and slightly superoinferiorly. The corresponding talar surface (a) also has this cylindrical shape with a similar radius and a similar axis, except that the surface of the talar cylinder is concave while that of the calcanean cylinder is convex.

As a whole the head of the talus is spherical and the bevelled surfaces on its circumference can be considered as facets chiselled out on a sphere (broken line) with centre g (fig. 6). Thus the anterior surface of the calcaneum (b) is biconcave while the corresponding talar surface is reciprocally biconvex. Very often the calcanean surface is indented in its middle and assumes the shape of the sole of a shoe; occasionally it is subdivided into two separate facets (figs. 7 and 8), one resting on the neck (b'_1) and the other on the sustentaculum tali (b'_2). It has been noted that the stability of the calcaneus is a function of the surface area of the latter facet. Occasionally the talus also presents two separate articular facets (b_1 and b_2).

The calcanean facet (b' or $b'_1 + b'_2$) is itself part of a much longer spherical surface which comprises in addition the posterior surface of the navicular (d)' and the upper edge of the plantar calcaneonavicular ligament (c'). With the help of the deltoid ligament (5) and the capsular ligament these surfaces form a spherical cavity which receives the head of the talus. On the head of the talus corresponding articular facets are present: the bulk of its articular surface (d) lodges into the navicular; between this (d) and the facet for the calcaneus (b) lies a triangular facet (c), which receives the calcaneonavicular ligament (c').

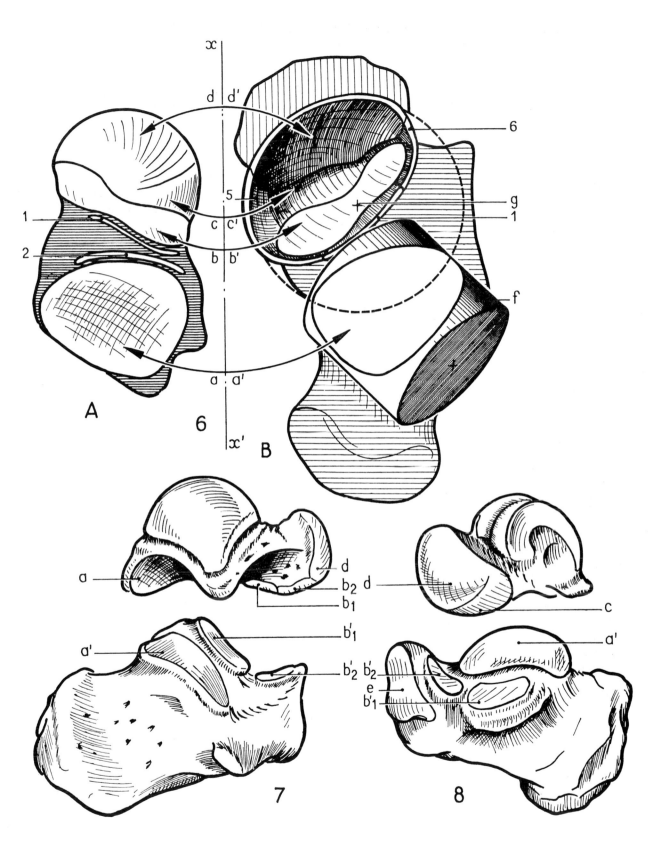

A

B

6

7

8

171

THE SUBTALAR JOINT: THE CONGRUENCE AND INCONGRUENCE OF THE ARTICULAR SURFACES

The description of the joint given on the previous page allows one to understand the orientation and the correspondence of the articular surfaces but not to grasp their peculiar modus operandi. For this purpose, the anterior subtalar joint must be described in greater detail. The opened joint is shown in figures 9 and 10 with the inferior aspect of the talus and the superior aspect of the anterior portion of the calcaneus (fig. 10). The numbers in the legends have the same meaning on the next page but are different from those on the previous page.

On the inferior aspect of the neck of the talus (fig. 9) the facet (b) corresponds to the facet (b'), lying on the superior aspect of the calcaneus (fig. 10), near the lateral tubercle. The head of the talus contains the articular surfaces for the navicular (e) and the distal tilia (d). The cartilage-lined surface, extending beyond the joint, is subdivided into **three facets** mediolaterally (C_1), (C_2) and (C_3), which correspond to the two facets (C'_1) and (C'_2) of the sustentculumtali (fig. 10). Posteriorly are seen the two surfaces of the posterior subtalar joint: the superior surface of the calcaneus (a') and the inferior surface of the talus (a).

There is only a **single position of articular congruence for the subtalar joint**, i.e. **the median position**. The foot is then straight without any inversion or eversion and it is the position adopted by a normal foot lying flat on a horizontal plane, in the resting position or during symmetrical double limb support. The articular surfaces of the posterior subtalar joint are not in perfect harmony. The facet (b) of the neck of the talus is in contact with the facet (b') on the neck of the calcaneus, while the middle facet (C_2) of the head of the talus is in contact with the horizontal facet (C'_1) of the sustentaculum tali. This neutral position, where the articular surfaces are kept together by the force of **gravity**, and not by the ligaments, is stable and can be maintained for a long time owing to the congruence of the articular surfaces. All other positions are **unstable** and are associated with a variable degree of articular **incongruence**.

During **eversion**, the anterior tip of the calcaneus (fig. 11: right side seen from above with a 'transparent' talus) is shifted laterally and tends to lie down (fig. 12: anterior view) on its medial surface. During this movement, the two facets (b) and (b') stay in contact forming a hinge, while the articular surface of the subtalar joint (a) slides inferiorly and anteriorly on the thalamus (a') to hit the floor of the sinus tarsi and the posterosuperior part of the thalamus is 'laid bare'. Anteriorly, the small talar fold (C_3) slides (fig. 12) on the surface of the oblique facet (C'_2) of the calcaneus. For this reason the two facets (C_2) and (C'_2) deserve the name of '**facets of eversion**'.

During **inversion** the calcaneus is displaced in the opposite direction with its anterior tip moving medially (fig. 13) and its lateral aspect tending to lie down flat (fig. 14). The two **hinge-facets** stay in contact, while the talar articular surface of the subtalar joint 'climbs' on the thalamus (a'), uncovering its anteroinferior aspect and anteriorly the **talar facet of inversion** (C_1) comes to rest on the horizontal facet (C'_1) of the sustentaculum tali (fig. 14).

These positions are therefore unstable with incongruent articular surfaces and are in the greatest need of ligamentous support. They can only be maintained **transiently**.

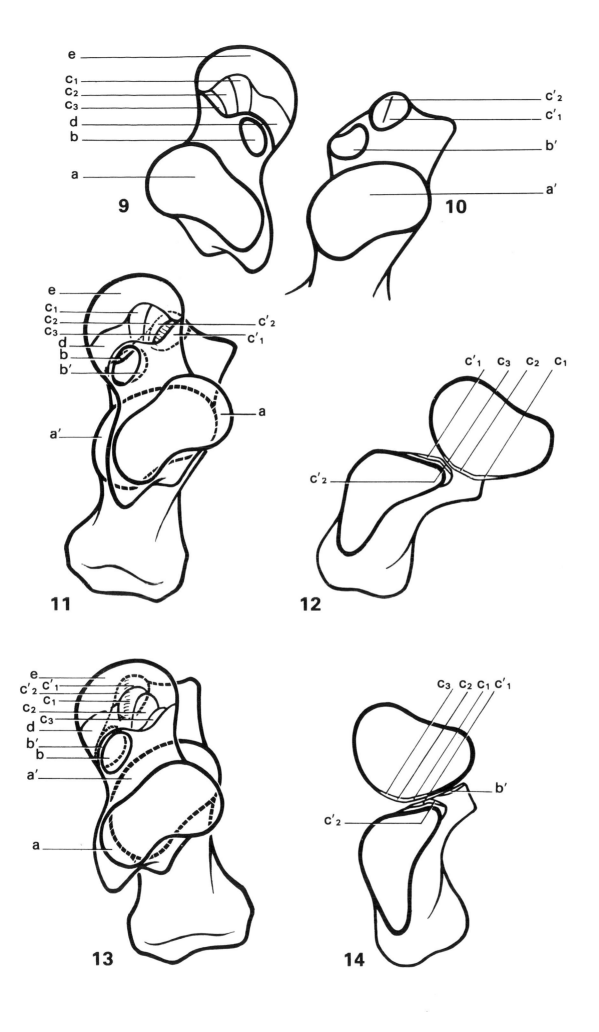

THE MOVEMENTS OF THE SUBTALAR JOINT

Taken separately each of the surfaces of the subtalar joint can be roughly approximated to a geometrical surface: the superior surface of the calcaneus is a segment of a cylinder, the head of the talus is a segment of a sphere. However, this joint must be considered to be a **plane joint**, because it is geometrically impossible for two spherical and two cylindrical surfaces (contained within a single mechanical joint) to slide simultaneously on one another without contact being lost between one of the sets of surfaces concerned. The joint possesses some measure of 'play' by virtue of its structure and stands in sharp contrast to a very tight joint (e.g. the hip joint), where the articular surfaces are geometrically congruent and allow minimal 'play'. If the surfaces of the subtalar joint are sufficiently congruent in the intermediate position, i.e. the position where the greatest degree of contact is required for support of the body weight, they become frankly *incongruent* in the extreme positions and the area of contact is reduced, but then the stresses on the joint are also reduced appreciably.

Starting from the intermediate position (fig. 29: the 'transparent' calcaneus and talus seen from inside), movements of the calcaneus on the talus (assumed to be fixed) occur **simultaneously in the three planes of space**. During **inversion of the foot** (p. 168) the anterior extremity of the calcaneus undergoes **three elementary movements** (fig. 30: initial position shown in dashes):

it moves slightly distally (t): slight extension of the foot;

it moves medially (v): adduction;

it comes to lie on the lateral surface (r): supination.

(The exact converse applies in the movement of eversion.)

Farabeuf has given the perfect description of this complex movement of the calcaneus: '*the calcaneus pitches, turns and rolls under the talus*'. This comparison to a ship is perfectly justified (fig. 33):

it pitches: its stem plunges into the waves (a);

it turns on itself (b);

it rolls by tilting to one side (c).

These elementary movements about the axes of pitching, turning and rolling are automatically fused as the ship dips obliquely into the wave (e).

It can be shown geometrically that a movement, whose elementary components about three axes are known, can be reduced to a *single movement occurring about a single axis* oblique to the three axes. In the case of the calcaneus, shown here diagrammatically as a paralleliped (fig. 31), this axis mn is olique supero-inferiorly, mediolaterally and anteroposteriorly. Rotation about this axis (fig. 32) results in the movements already described. This axis, demonstrated by Henke, enters at the superomedial aspect of the talar neck, runs through the sinus tarsi and emerges at the posterolateral tubercle of the calcaneus (p. 186). The axis of Henke not only applies to the subtalar joint but also to the transverse tarsal joint. Therefore it controls all the movements of the posterior tarsus underneath the ankle.

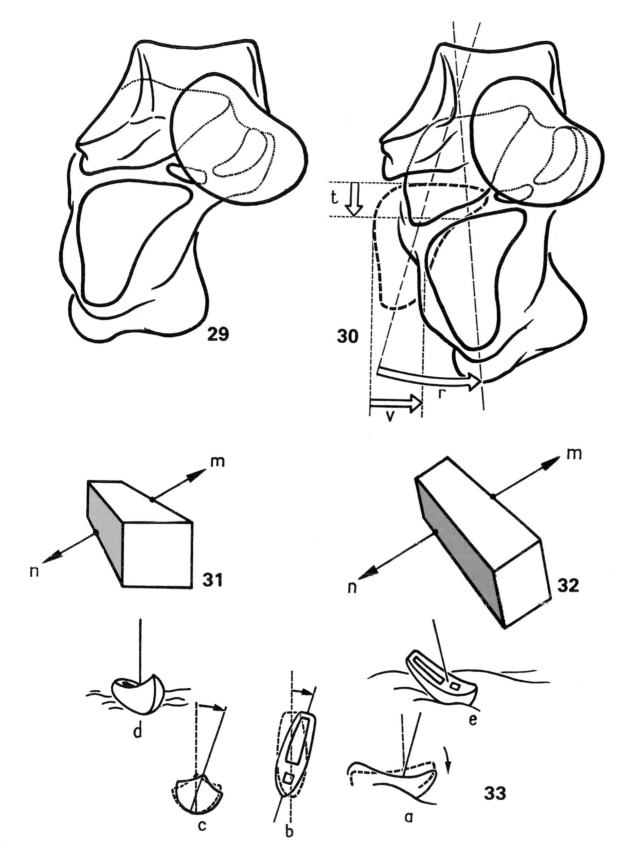

29

30

t

v

r

m

n

31

m

n

32

d

c

b

a

e

33

181

THE MOVEMENTS OF THE SUBTALAR AND TRANSVERSE TARSAL JOINTS

The relative displacements of the bones of the posterior tarsus are easily analysed with the use of an anatomical preparation and skiagrams taken in the positions of inversion and eversion. If each bone is transfixed with a metal pin (a: for the talus; b: for the calcaneus; c: for the navicular; d: for the cuboid) the angular displacements can be calculated.

On a **radiograph taken vertically** (seen from above), the calcaneus staying put, the change from eversion (fig. 34) to inversion (fig. 35) is associated with the following displacements:

the navicular (c) slides medially on the talar head and turns through an angle of 5°;

the cuboid (a) follows the navicular and turns through the same angle and slides medially relative to the calcaneus and the navicular;

the calcaneus (b) moves anteriorly slightly and turns on the talus through an angle of 5°.

These three elementary rotations occur in the same direction, i.e. in *adduction*.

An **anteroposterior radiograph**, the talus being taken to be stationary, shows the following displacement during change from eversion (fig. 36) to inversion (fig. 37):

the navicular (c) turns through an angle of 25° and 'overflows' the talus medially;

the cuboid (d) is completely lost behind the shadow of the calcaneus and turns through an angle of 18°;

the calcaneus (b) slides medially under the talus and turns through an angle of 20°.

These three elementary rotations occur in the same direction i.e. that of *supination*, and the navicular turns more than the calcaneus and especially more than the cuboid.

Finally, on **a lateral view**, during change from eversion (fig. 38) to inversion (fig. 39) the following displacements are noted:

The navicular (b) literally slides under the talar head and turns on itself through an angle of 45° so that its anterior surface tends to face inferiorly.

The cuboid (d) also slides inferiorly in relation to both the calcaneus and the talus; this inferior movement of the cuboid with respect to the talus is distinctly more important than that of the navicular relative to the talus. At the same time the cuboid turns through an angle of 12°.

The calcaneus (b) finally moves anteriorly relative to the talus so that the posterior edge of the talus comes to overhang the part of the calcaneus lying posterior to its superior articular facet. At the same time it turns through an angle of 12° in the direction of extension, like the navicular.

These three elementary movements occur in the same direction, i.e. that of extension.

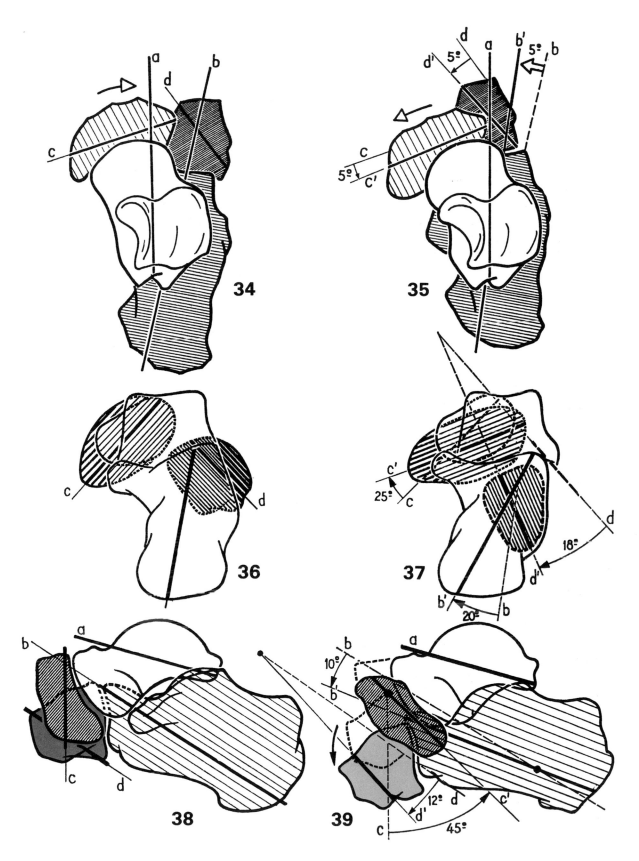

THE MOVEMENTS OF THE TRANSVERSE TARSAL JOINT

These movements depend on the shape of the articular surfaces and the arrangement of the ligaments.

Taken as a whole, (fig. 40) the articular surfaces are set in relation to an axis xx′ which runs obliquely supero-inferiorly and lateromedially at an angle of 45° with the horizontal. It serves as a '*hinge*' which allows the navicular and the cuboid to move inferiorly and medially (arrows S and C) or superiorly and laterally. The surface of the talar head, which is oval with its great axis yy′ inclined at an angle of 45° with the horizontal (the angle of 'rotation' of the talus), is longer in the direction of this movement.

The displacements of the navicular on the head of the talus take place medially (fig. 41) and inferiorly (fig. 42) under the pull of the tibialis posterior (TP) which is inserted into the tubercle of the navicular. The tension of the dorsal talonavicular ligament (a) checks these movements. This change in the direction of the navicular produces, via the cuneiform bones and the first three metatarsals, adduction and hollowing of the medial plantar arch (p. 220).

At the same time **the navicular moves relative to the calcaneus**. In the *position of eversion* (fig. 43: seen from above; the talus has been removed) the 'spring' ligament (b), the lower edge of the deltoid ligament (c) and the medial band of the bifurcated ligament (d) are under tension; *when the foot is inverted* (fig. 44), contraction of the tibialis posterior (TP) brings the navicular closer to the calcaneus and makes the talus move up the superior surface of the calcaneus (striped arrow) so that the above-mentioned ligaments are relaxed. This explains why the anterior surface of the calcaneus does not extend as far down as the navicular: an articular surface, supported by a bony bracket, and consequently rigid, would not allow these displacements of the navicular relative to the calcaneus. On the other hand, the flexible surface of the spring ligament (b) is essential (p. 220) for the elasticity of the medial arch of the foot.

The superior movements of the cuboid on the calcaneus (fig. 45: seen from the medial aspect) are severely limited by two factors:

the anterior process of the calcaneus (arrow) which constitutes an obstacle on the proximal side of the transverse tarsal joint;

the tension of the powerful plantar calcaneocuboid ligament (f) which rapidly stops the interspace of the joint (α) from opening out inferiorly.

On the other hand, inferior movement of the cuboid (fig. 46) easily takes place over the convexity of the articular facet of the calcaneus; it is only checked by tension of the lateral band (e) of the bifurcated ligament.

In the transverse plane (fig. 47: horizontal section at the level AB of fig. 40) the cuboid glides more easily medially being checked by tension of the dorsal calcaneocuboid ligament (g). Taken as a whole, displacement of the cuboid takes place preferentially *inferiorly and medially*.

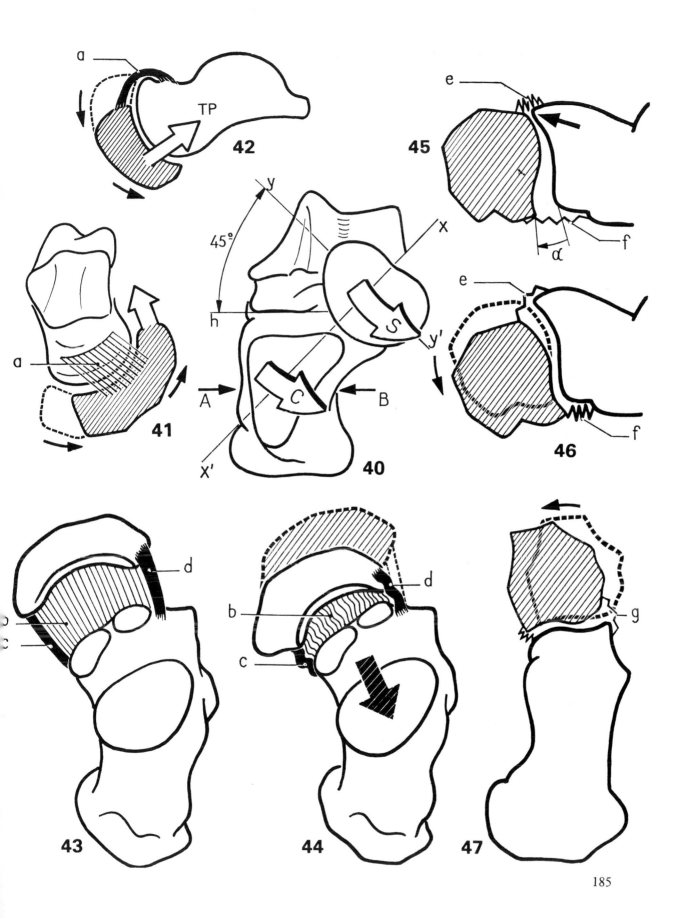

THE OVERALL FUNCTION OF THE JOINTS OF THE POSTERIOR TARSUS
(The legends are the same as those of p. 178.)

It is clear from examining and manipulating an anatomical preparation of the posterior part of the foot that all these joints constitute an inseparable functional unit, *the articular complex of the posterior tarsus*, concerned with altering the direction and shape of the arches of the foot. The subtalar and the transverse tarsal joints are mechanically linked and together form a single joint with **one degree of freedom** about the axis of Henke (mn).

The diagrams show the four bones of the posterior part of the foot from two different angles: two different perspectives, anterolateral (figs. 48 and 50) and anterior (figs. 49 and 51). In these diagrams the positions corresponding to inversion (figs. 48 and 49) and those corresponding to eversion (figs. 50 and 51) are correspondingly arranged one above the other. This makes it easier to appreciate the changes in direction of the navicular and cuboid bones relative to the talus, which by definition stays put.

Movement of inversion (figs. 48 and 49):

the tibialis posterior pulls on the navicular (nav) exposing the superolateral part of the talar head (d);

the navicular drags the cuboid along via the cubonavicular ligaments;

the cuboid in turn pulls on the calcaneus (Calc) which moves anteriorly under the talus (Tal);

the sinus tarsi opens to its widest (fig. 48) while the two bands of the interosseous ligament (1 and 2) are stretched;

the superior articular facet of the calcaneus (a') is laid bare on its antero-inferior aspect while the interspace of the subtalar joint gapes open superoposteriorly.

Taken as a whole:

the navicular and cuboid bones together are drawn medially (fig. 49: arrow Add) so that the forefoot *moves anteriorly and medially* (arrow I, fig. 48).

At the same time *the pair scaphoid-cuboid turns round an anteroposterior axis running through the bifurcated ligament*, which actively resists stresses of torsion and traction. This rotation, due to the superior displacement of the scaphoid and the inferior movement of the cuboid, produces **supination** (arrow Supin): the sole of the foot faces medially because the lateral plantar arch is lowered—the articular facet of the cuboid, corresponding to the base of the fifth metatarsal (Vm) faces anteriorly and inferiorly—while the medial arch is elevated—the articular facet of the navicular for the medial cuneiform (Ic) moves anteriorly.

Movement of eversion (figs. 50 and 51):

the peroneus brevis, inserted into the tuberosity of the base of the fifth metatarsal, pulls the cuboid laterally and posteriorly;

the cuboid draws the navicular along so that the superomedial part of the talar head is exposed;

the calcaneus is also drawn along and moves posteriorly under the talus;

the sinus tarsi closes down (fig. 50) and the movement of eversion is checked by impact of the talus on to the floor of the sinus tarsi;

the posterosuperior part of the superior surface of the calcaneus (a') is uncovered.

Taken as a whole:

the navicular and cuboid bones (fig. 51) together are pulled laterally (arrow Abd) so that the forefoot is drawn *anteriorly and laterally* (arrow E, fig. 50).

At the same time it rotates in the direction of **pronation** (arrow Pron) as a result of inferior displacement of the navicular and abduction of the cuboid so that its articular facet for the fifth metatarsal (Vm) looks anteriorly and laterally.

186

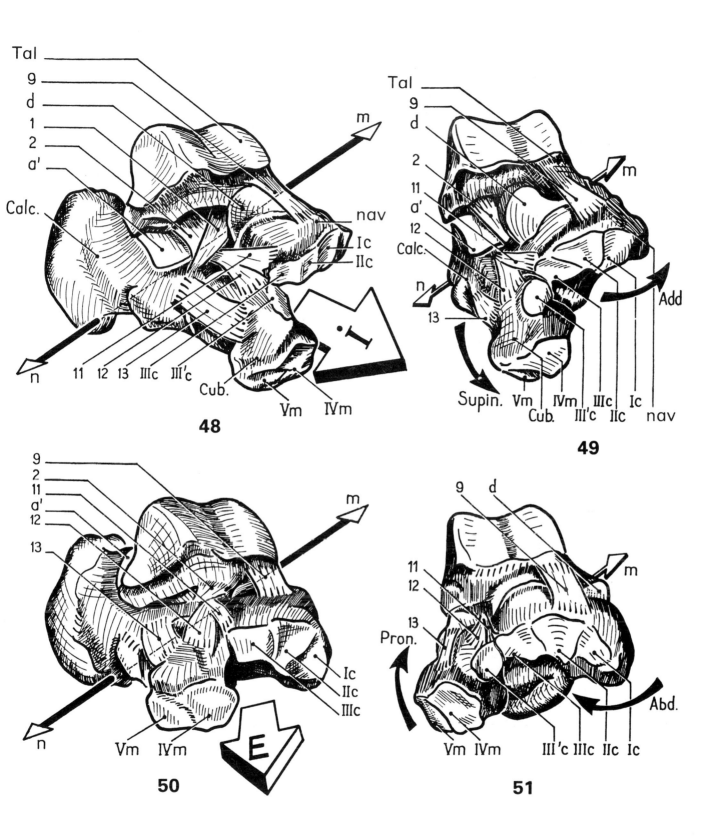

Tal
9
d
1
2
a'
Calc.
m
nav
Ic
IIc
n
11 12 13 IIIc III'c
Cub.
Vm IVm

48

Tal
9
d
2
11
a'
12
Calc.
m
n
13
Add
Supin. Vm IVm IIIc Ic
Cub. III'c IIc nav

49

9
2
11
a'
12
13
m
n
Vm IVm
Ic
IIc
IIIc

E

50

9 d
11
12
13
m
Pron.
Abd.
Vm IVm III'c IIIc IIc Ic

51

187

THE HETEROKINETIC UNIVERSAL JOINT OF THE POSTERIOR TARSUS

Henke's axis is not, as one might think, fixed and unchanging. In fact it is a **changing axis**, i.e. shifting in space during movements. This conclusion can be drawn from successive radiographs of the posterior tarsus taken during inversion and eversion. If one superimposes the instantaneous centres of rotation identified on corresponding radiographs, *they do not coincide*. This observation justifies the hypothesis that Henke's axis (fig. 52) moves from an initial (1) to a final (2) position, describing a 'crooked path' between these extreme positions. The mathematical demonstration of this hypothesis on computer remains to be done.

In the posterior tarsus, there are **two successive non-parallel axes**, the axis of the ankle and Henke's axis, which can be viewed as the global axis of the subtalar and transverse tarsal joints. It is thus justifiable to use the **universal joint** as the mechanical model of the *articular complex of the posterior tarsus*.

In **mechanics** the universal joint is defined as a joint with two axes perpendicular to each other and comprising two forks (fig. 53), which can rotate one on the other at any angle. In cars with frontwheel drive it is inserted between the driving shaft and the axle. It is known as the 'homokinetic universal joint' because the rotational couple of force is always the same regardless of the relative positions of the forks.

In **biomechanics**, there are *three joints* of this type:

the sternoclavicular joint—a saddle joint;

the wrist—a condyloid joint;

the trapezometacarpal joint—a saddle joint, studied in detail in volume I.

In the posterior tarsus the articular complex consists of a **'heterokinetic' universal joint**. Its axes are not orthogonal, i.e. perpendicular to each other in space, but are *oblique*. A mechanical model is provided in figure 54, where the following structures can be seen:

the leg (A) and the forefoot (B);

the transverse axis xx' of the ankle, running obliquely anteriorly and medially;

Henke's axis, running obliquely in a posteroanterior, inferosuperior and lateromedial direction;

an intervening piece (C), which has no bony equivalent but which represents a distorted tetrahedron with the two axes of the universal joint running through two of its corners.

The relative obliquity of these two non-orthogonal axes gives rise to a **directional bias** in the movements of the posterior tarsus. The muscles, distributed about these two axes (p. 235), can only produce **two types of movement** (*with other types of movement being 'prohibited'*):

inversion (fig. 55), which extends the foot and turns the plantar surface to face medially;

eversion (fig. 56), which flexes the foot and turns the plantar surface to face laterally.

A grasp of this 'heterokinetic universal joint' is basic to our understanding of the actions of the muscles of the foot, the orientation of the plantar surface of the foot as well as the static and dynamic functions of the foot.

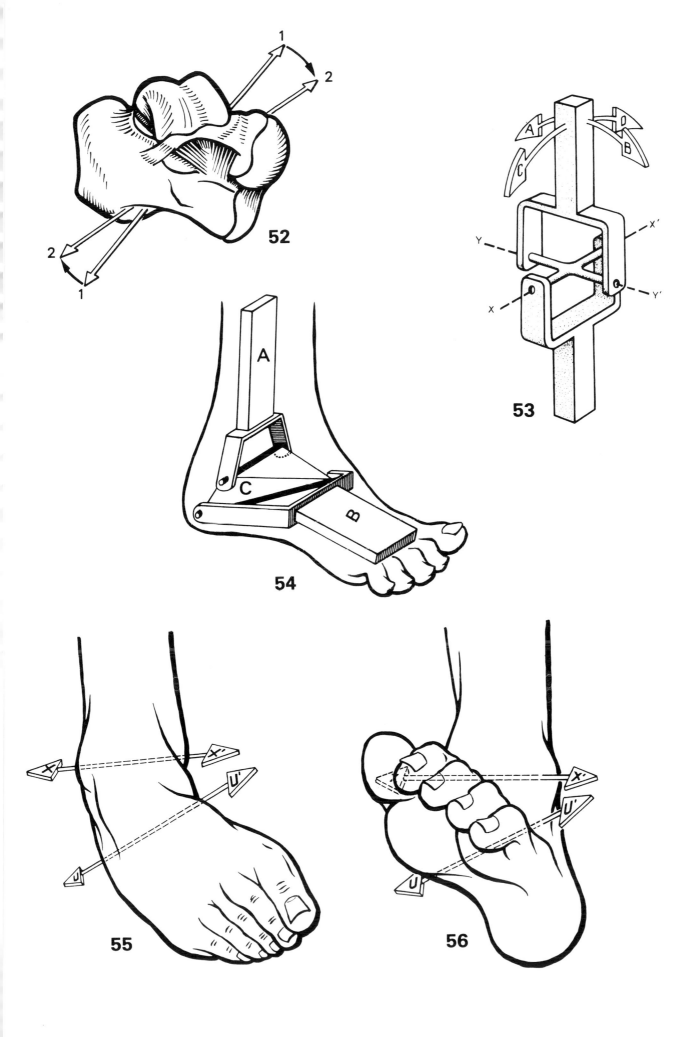

52

53

54

55

56

MOVEMENTS OF THE ANTERIOR TARSAL AND TARSOMETATARSAL JOINTS

The **intercuneiform joints** (fig. 65: frontal section) allow small vertical movements to occur which alter the curvature of the transverse plantar arch (p. 226). The lateral cuneiform (C_l) rests on the cuboid (Cub) whose medial third (striped) provides support for the cuneiform arch.

Slight displacements of the cuneiforms relative to the navicular (nav) occur along the long axis of the foot (fig. 66: sagittal section) and contribute to the changes of curvature of the medial arch (p. 220).

The movements of the tarsometatarsal joints (can be deduced from their anatomical features, especially the shape of the joint interspaces and the orientation of the articular surfaces (fig. 67: seen from above):

As a whole the line of the tarsometatarsal joints runs *obliquely mediolaterally, supero-inferiorly* and *anteroposteriorly*. Its medial end lies 2 cm. anterior to its lateral end. The general obliquity of this axis of flexion and extension of the tarsometatarsal joints contributes, just as the obliquity of the axis of Henke, to the movements of eversion and inversion.

The distances by which the cuneiforms overstep one another and the cuboid are in geometric progression:

the lateral cuneiform (C_l) oversteps the cuboid (Cub) by 2 mm.;

the lateral cuneiform (C_l) oversteps the intermediate cuneiform (C_i) by 4 mm.;

the medial cuneiform (Cm) oversteps the intermediate cuneiform by 8 mm.

Thus is constituted the deep mortise which lodges the base of the second metatarsal. This metatarsal is therefore the least mobile and forms the crest-tile of the plantar arches (p. 224).

The two end segments of this line of the metatarsal joints have the opposite oliquity:

The interspace of the first metatarso-medial cuneiform joint is oblique anteriorly and *laterally* and, when produced, it runs through the middle of the fifth metatarsal; the interspace of the fifth metatarsocuboid joint is oblique anteriorly and *medially* and, when produced, runs almost through the head of the first metatarsal.

Therefore the axis of flexion and extension of the lateral metatarsals, which are the most mobile, is not perpendicular but oblique to their long axes. So these metatarsals do not move in a sagittal plane but over the segment of a cone: during flexion they also move towards the axis of the foot (fig. 69: schematic superotateral view of tarsometatarsal joint line with the first and fifth metatarsals included):

the movement aa' of the head of M_I is compounded of a movement of flexion (F) and one of abduction (Abd), which has a range of 15° (Fick);

conversely, the movement bb' of the head of M_V is compounded of a movement of flexion (F) and one of adduction (Add).

Therefore the heads of these metatarsals not only move inferiorly but also towards the axis of the foot and this **increases** (fig. 70) **the curvature of the anterior arch** with hollowing of the anterior part of the foot. Conversely, extension of the metatarsals is followed by flattening of the arch.

This approximation of the lateral metatarsals is also assisted (fig. 68: the articular surfaces of the cuboid and cuneiforms seen from the front) by the obliquity of the transverse axes (xx' and yy') of their articular surfaces. This movement occurs along the thick double-headed arrows.

Therefore changes in the curvature of the anterior arch result from movements occurring at the tarsometatarsal joints.

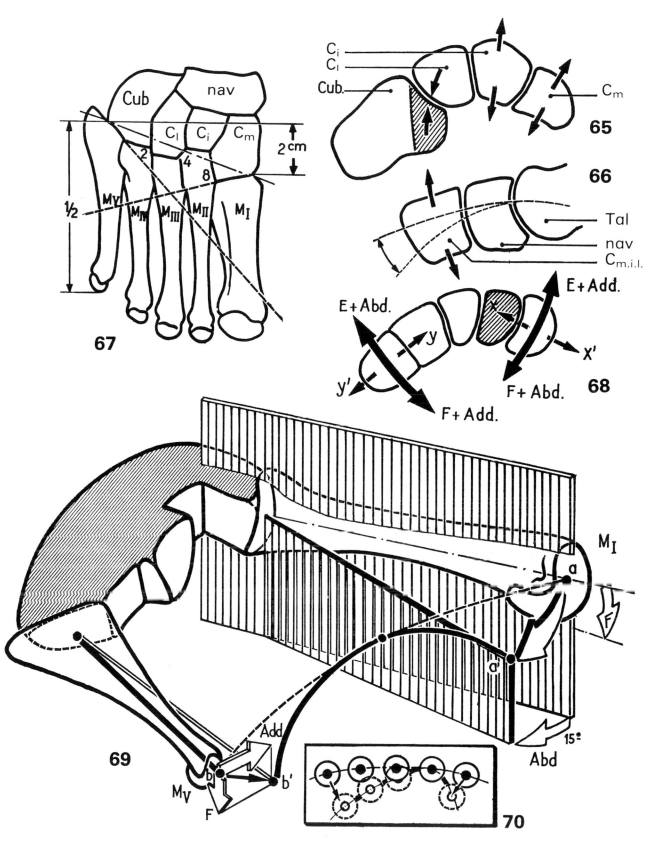

65

66

67

68

E+Add.

E+Abd.

F+Abd.

F+Add.

Tal

nav

$C_{m.i.l.}$

C_i
C_l
Cub.

C_m

Cub   nav

C_l C_i C_m

2 cm

½ M_V

M_{IV} M_{III} M_{II} M_I

2   4   8

M_I

F

15°

Abd

69

Add

M_V

b   b'

F

70

a

a'

195

EXTENSION OF THE TOES

The metatarsophalangeal and interphalangeal joints will not be described as they are identical to those of the fingers (see Vol. I), except for some functional differences. Thus, whereas at the metacarpophalangeal joints flexion has a greater range than extension, extension **exceeds** flexion at the metatarsophalangeal joints:

active extension has a range of 50° to 60°, active flexion only 30° to 40°;

passive extension, which is essential in the final phase of taking a step (fig. 71), reaches or exceeds 90° while passive flexion has a range of 45° to 50°.

Side-to-side movements of the toes occur at the metatarsophalangeal joints and have a far smaller range than those of the fingers. In particular man's big toe, in contrast to that of the monkey, has lost all *movement of opposition* during adaptation to walking on two legs.

Active extension of the toes is produced by *three muscles*: two extrinsic muscles—the extensor hallucis longus and extensor digitorum longus—and one intrinsic muscle—extensor digitorum brevis.

The **extensor digitorum brevis** (fig. 72) lies entirely in the dorsum of the foot. It arises from the sulcus calcanei (i.e. the floor of the sinus tarsi) and from the stem of the inferior extensor retinaculum. It divides into four fleshy bellies which are inserted by tendon into the lateral sides of the corresponding tendons of the extensor digitorum longus, except for the tendon (destined for the first metatarsal), which is inserted directly into the dorsal surface of first phalanx of the big toe; the fifth toe receives no tendon from this muscle. Therefore the extensor digitorum brevis is an extensor of the metatarsophalangeal joints of the first four toes (fig. 73).

The extensor digitorum longus and the extensor hallucis longus are lodged in the anterior compartment of the leg; their tendons terminate on the phalanges (see p. 198).

The extensor digitorum longus (fig. 74) runs anterior to the ankle deep to the lateral half of the superior extensor retinaculum and then passes posterior to the stem of the inferior extensor retinaculum before dividing into four tendons which run to the four lesser toes. Therefore the fifth toe is only extended by the extensor digitorum longus. This muscle, as its name indicates, is an extensor of the toes but it is *also and above all* (p. 204) *a flexor of the ankle*. Its primary action on the toes is only apparent when its flexor action on the ankle is counterbalanced by the antagonistic extensor of the ankle (the Achilles tendon is shown as an arrow).

The **tendon of the extensor hallucis longus** (fig. 75) runs deep to the superior extensor retinaculum and then pierces the two limbs of the inferior extensor retinaculum. It is inserted into the dorsal aspect of the two phalanges of the big toe: on the two borders of the dorsum of the first phalanx and the dorsal aspect of the base of the terminal phalax. It is therefore an extensor of the big toe but *also and above all a flexor of the ankle*. As with the extensor digitorum longus, its primary action on the big toe is only apparent when its flexor action on the ankle is cancelled by the antagonistic extensors of the ankle.

Duchenne de Boulogne claims that the extensor digitorum brevis is the only true extensor of the toes; this claim will be justified later.

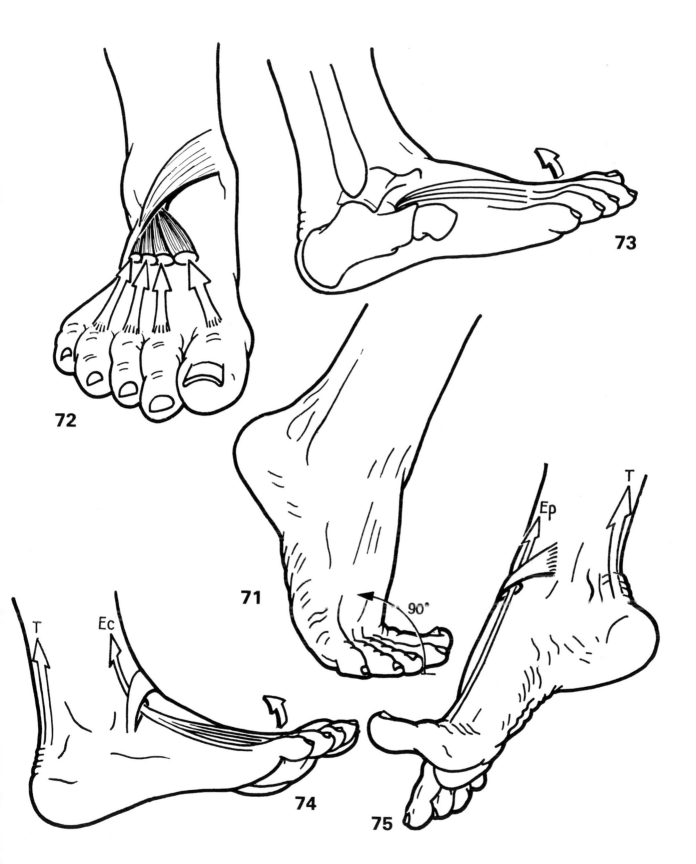

72

73

71

74

75

197

THE INTEROSSEOUS AND THE LUMBRICAL MUSCLES
(the numbers have the same meaning in all the diagrams).

As in the hand, the interossei fall into two groups—dorsal and plantar—but their arrangement is slightly different in the foot (fig. 76: frontal section of the foot, posterior slice shown). The **four dorsal interossei** (Ix. d) are, as it were, centred on the second metatarsal (instead of the third as in the hand) and are inserted into the second toe and the two immediately adjacent toes (fig. 83: white arrows). The **three plantar interossei** (Ix. p) arise from the medial aspect of the plantar surfaces of the last three metatarsals and are inserted into the corresponding toe (fig. 84).

The mode of insertion of the interossei of the foot is similar to that of the interossei of the hand (fig. 77: dorsal view of the extensor tendons; fig. 79: side view of the muscles of the toes):

they are inserted into the medial or lateral side of the first phalanges (1);

they are also attached to the collateral digital expansions (3) of the extensor tendons by a tendinous expansion (2).

The tendon of the extensor digitorum longus (EDL) is inserted into the toes just as the extensor digitorum communis is into the fingers:

by some fibres (4) into the borders of the first phalanx (P_1) and not into its base;

by a median dorsal expansion (5) into the base of P_2;

by two collateral expansions (3) into the base of P_3.

Proximal to the first metatarsophalangeal joint (fig. 78: dorsal view) the tendons of the extensor digitorum longus for the second, third and fourth toes receive the corresponding tendons from the extensor digitorum brevis (EDB).

As in the hand, there are **four lumbricals** (figs. 76, 78 and 88) arising from the tendons of the flexor digitorum longus (the homologue of flexor digitorum profundus of the hand). Each lumbrical runs *medially* (fig. 88) to be inserted (figs. 78 and 79) like an interosseus, i.e. into the base of P_1 (6) and into the collateral expansion of the extensor longus (7).

The **tendon of the flexor digitorum longus** (FDL), like the flexor digitorum profundus in the hand (figs. 79 and 88), runs against the fibrocartilaginous plate (8) of the first metatarsophalangeal joint, and then 'perforates' the tendon of the flexor digitorum brevis (FDB) before gaining insertion into the base of the distal phalanx. The flexor digitorum brevis is therefore analogous to the flexor digitorum sublimis: it is superficial and its tendon is '*perforated*' by the tendon of the long flexor prior to its insertion into the margins of the second phalanx. Thus the flexor digitorum longus flexes the distal interphalangeal joint (fig. 81), while the flexor digitorum brevis flexes the proximal interphalangeal joint. The interossei and lumbrical muscles, as in the hand, flex the metatarsophalangeal joint (fig. 80) and extend the interphalangeal joints. They play a vital part in the stabilisation of the toes: by flexing the metatarsophalangeal joint they provide a strong point of attachment for the extensors of the toes as they flex the ankle. When the interossei and lumbricals are paralysed a 'claw foot' (fig. 82) can result: as the metatarsophalangeal joint is no longer stabilised by the interossei, it is hyperextended by the extensors and the phalanx slides over the dorsal surface of the head of the metatarsal. The foot is then secondarily fixed in this abnormal position by the dorsal displacement of the interossei above the axis (+) of the metatarsophalangeal joint. Furthermore the interphalangeal joints are flexed as a result of the 'relative shortening' of the flexors and this is followed by dorsal subluxation of the proximal interphalangeal joint (black arrow) between the collateral expansions of the extensor tendon so that the action of the extensor is now reversed.

As in the hand, the position of the toes depends therefore on the balance struck among different muscles. Thus it becomes apparent, as claims Duchenne de Boulogne, that only the extensor digitorum brevis is the true extensor of the toes; the extensors are in actual fact flexors of the ankle and so, according to Duchenne, would be more 'efficient' if they were inserted directly into the metatarsals.

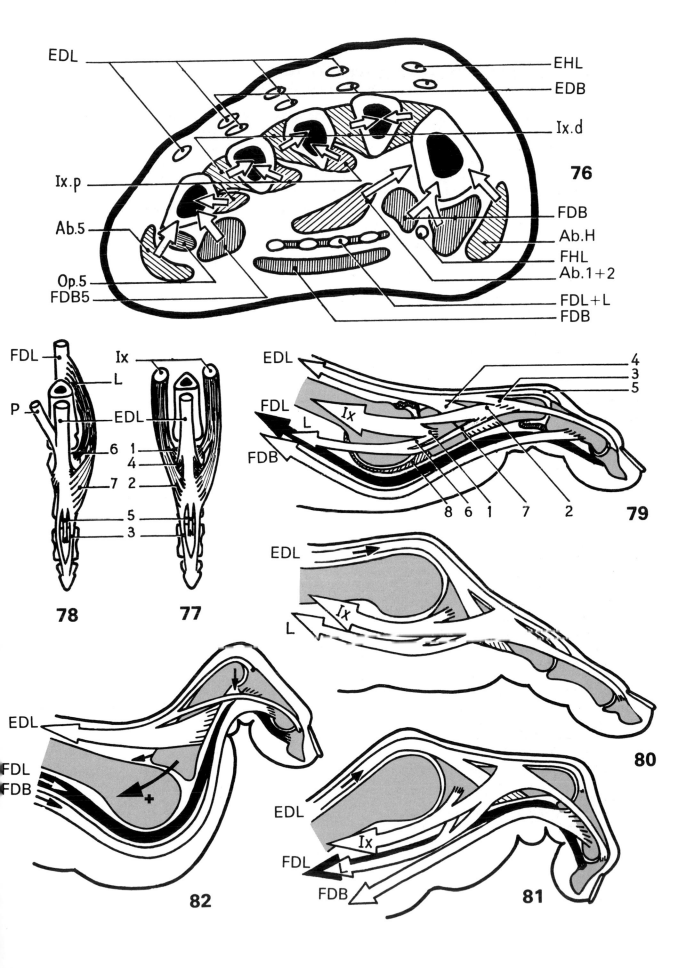

EDL

EHL

EDB

Ix.d

76

Ix.p

FDB

Ab.5

Ab.H

FHL

Op.5

Ab.1+2

FDB5

FDL+L

FDB

FDL

Ix

L

P

EDL

6 1

4

7 2

5

3

78

77

EDL

4

3

5

FDL

Ix

L

FDB

8 6 1 7 2

79

EDL

Ix

L

80

EDL

FDL

FDB

82

EDL

Ix

FDL

FDB

81

THE SOLE OF THE FOOT: THE PLANTAR MUSCLES

(the numbers and letters have the same meaning as in the diagrams of the previous page).

A. The **deep layer** consists of the interossei and the muscles attached to the fifth toe and to the big toe:

The dorsal interossei (fig. 83: seen from below), in addition to being flexors and extensors of the toes, also abduct the toes away from the axis of the foot (second metatarsal and second toe). The big toe is 'abducted' by the abductor hallucis (Ab. H) and the little toe by the abductor digiti minimi (Ab. 5). These two muscles are therefore *analogous to dorsal interossei*.

The plantar interossei (fig. 84: seen from below) move the last three toes closer to the second toe. The big toe is adducted by the adductor hallucis which consists of two heads:

the oblique head (Ad. 1) which arises from the bones of the anterior tarsus;

the transverse head (Ad. 2) which arises from the plantar ligaments of the third, fourth and fifth metatarsophalangeal joints and from the deep transverse ligaments. It draws the first phalanx of the big toe directly laterally and plays a part in supporting the anterior arch (p. 224).

The muscles of the fifth toe (fig. 85: seen from below) are three in number and lie within the lateral compartment of the foot:

the *opponens digiti minimi* (Op. 5) is the deepest of these muscles: it runs from the anterior tarsus to the fifth metatarsal and has a similar action to that of the opponens of the fifth finger but is less efficient. It hollows the lateral arch and the anterior arch.

The other two muscles are both inserted into the lateral side of the base of the first phalanx, i.e. the *flexor digiti minimi brevis* (FDB 5) which takes origin from the anterior tarsus and the *abductor digiti minimi* (Ab. 5), which arises (fig. 86) from the posterolateral tubercle of the calcaneus and the tuberosity of the fifth metatarsal and assists in the maintenance of the lateral arch (p. 222).

The muscles of the big toe (fig. 85) are three in number and lie in the medial compartment of the foot (except for the adductor). They are inserted into the lateral aspect of the base of the first phalanx and into the two sesamoid bones articulating with the head of the first metatarsal.

On the medial side a sesamoid and the first phalanx give insertion to *the medial portion of the flexor hallucis brevis* (FHB) and to the *abductor hallucis* (Ab. H) which arises from the posteromedial tubercle of the calcaneus (fig. 86) and assists in the support of the medial arch (p. 222).

On the lateral side, a sesamoid bone and the first phalanx receive the insertion of the *two heads of the adductor hallucis* (Ad. 1 and 2) and of *the lateral portion of the flexor hallucis brevis* (FHB), which arises from the bones of the anterior tarsus.

These muscles are powerful flexors of the big toe: they play an important part in stabilisation of the big toe and in the last phase of the step (p. 230). Their paralysis leads to a 'claw' deformity of the big toe.

B. **The intermediate layer** consists of the long flexor muscles (fig. 87). **The flexor digitorum longus** (FDL) crosses the flexor hallucis longus (FHL) from below as they emerge from under the sustentaculum tali and receives from it a strong tendinous slip (9). It then divides into four tendons for the four lesser toes. The lumbricals (fig. 88) take origin from two contiguous tendons, except the first lumbrical (4). The obliquity of the pull of these tendons is compensated by a flat muscle which runs along the long axis of the sole of the foot: it arises from the posteromedial and posterolateral tubercles of the calcaneus and is inserted into the lateral border of the tendon for the little toe (fig. 87). By contracting simultaneously, this muscle—the flexor digitorum accessorius (FDA)—decreases the obliquity of these tendons relative to the axis of the foot.

The **flexor hallucis longus** (FHL, figs. 85 and 87) runs in a groove between the two sesamoid bones embedded in the flexor hallucis brevis and gains insertion into the distal phalanx of the big toe.

C. **The superficial layer** consists of a single muscle (fig. 86), which lies in the middle plantar compartment. It is **the flexor digitorum brevis** (FDB), which arises from the posteromedial and posterolateral tubercles of the calcaneus and is inserted by tendon into the middle phalanges of the four lesser toes. It is analogous to the flexor digitorum sublimis of the hand: its tendons are '*perforated*' (fig. 88) and are inserted into the middle phalanx which they flex.

200

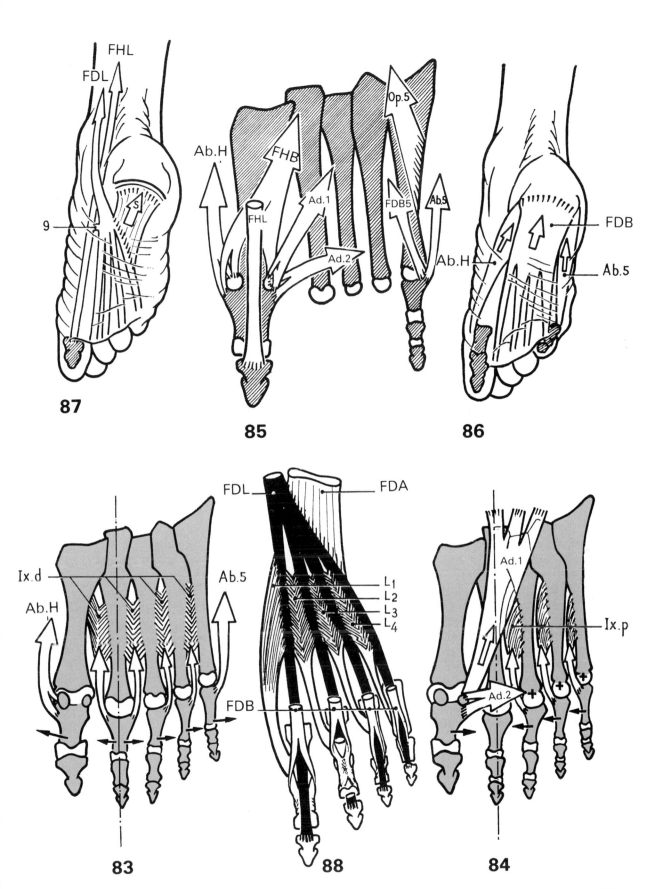

87

85

86

83

88

84

201

THE FIBROUS TUNNELS OF THE DORSAL AND PLANTAR ASPECTS OF THE FOOT

The **inferior extensor retinaculum** (fig. 89) keeps the four dorsal tendons of the foot pressed against the tarsal bones at the level of the concavity of the instep: thus it acts as the hinge of a pulley for these tendons whatever the degree of flexion of the ankle. It arises from the superior surface of the calcaneus in front of the sulcus calcanei and soon divides into two diverging bands:

an **inferior band** (a), which blends with the deep fascia of the medial border of the foot;

a **superior band** (b) which is attached to the anterior margin of the tibia near the medial malleolus. This band consists in turn of *distinct lambellae*:

medially, the deep and superficial lamellae embrace the tendon of the tibialis anterior (TA) which is invested in a synovial sheath starting two fingers' breadth proximal to the retinaculum;

laterally these two lamellae form two separate fibrous loops: the medial loop lodges the tendon of the extensor hallucis longus (EHL), invested in a synovial sheath which barely overlaps the retinaculum proximally; the lateral loop contains the tendons of extensor digitorum longus (EDL) and of the peroneus tertisu (P.T.), invested in a common synovial sheath which starts slightly above the retinaculum.

All the other tendons pass through tunnels which lie behind the malleoli.

Posterior to the lateral malleolus (fig. 90) the tendons of the peroneus brevis (PB) and of the peroneus longus (PL) run in an osteofibrous tunnel (1) bounded by the fibula and the superior peroneal retinaculum. These tendons are parallel, with the former lying posterior and inferior to the latter. They bend sharply anteriorly below the malleolar tip and are tethered in two osteofibrous tunnels (3 and 4), bounded by the lateral aspect of the calcaneus, the peroneal tubercle (5) and the inferior peroneal retinaculum. At this point their common synovial sheath divides into two separate sheaths. This peroneus brevis (PB) is inserted into the lateral tubercle of the base of the M_V and the base of the M_{IV}. A small segment (7) of this tendon has been resected to display the tendon of the peroneus longus as it changes its direction and enters the groove on the undersurface of the cuboid. The peroneus longus, invested by a new synovial sheath, then runs on the plantar aspect of the foot (fig. 91) through an osteofibrous tunnel constituted superiorly by the tarsal bones and inferiorly by the superficial fibres of the long plantar ligament (fig. 91: deep fibres, 8), which runs from the calcaneus (9) to the cuboid and thence to the bases of all the metatarsals (x), and by fibres of the terminal expansion of the tibialis posterior tendon (TP). The tendon of peroneus longus is inserted mainly into the base of the first metatarsal (11) but also by expansions into the second metatarsal and the medial cuneiform. As it enters the plantar tunnel it is associated almost regularly with a sesamoid bone (12) which allows the tendon to alter its direction more easily.

Therefore the plantar aspect of the foot is carpeted by three sets of fibrous expansions:

the longitudinal fibres of the long plantar ligament;

the fibres of the tendon of the peroneus longus running obliquely anteriorly and medially;

the fibrous expansions of the tibialis posterior tendon which run obliquely anteriorly and laterally to all the tarsal and metatarsal bones, except the last two metatarsals.

Posterior to the medial malleolus (fig. 92) run three tendons which are contained in an osteofibrous tunnel, formed by the tibia and the flexor retinaculum, and are invested in separate synovial sheaths. These tendons are arranged anteroposteriorly and mediolaterally as follows:

The **tibialis posterior** (TP) runs close to the malleolus and bends sharply anteriorly at its tip to gain insertion into the tuberosity of the navicular bone (14) while sending numerous fibrous slips to the plantar aspect of the tarsal and metatarsal bones (10).

The **flexor digitorum longus** (FDL) runs close to the tibialis posterior and along the inner surface of the sustentaculum tali (15; see also fig. 94). It then crosses the deep surface (16) of the flexor hallucis longus.

The **flexor hallucis longus** (FHL) crosses between the posteromedial and posterolateral tubercles (17) of the talus (p. 156) and then below the sustentaculum tali (18; see also fig. 94). Therefore it changes its direction twice.

Two coronal sections (right foot), taken at levels A and B given in figures 90 and 92, illustrate the arrangement of these tendons and of their synovial sheaths in the retromalleolar tunnels: section A (fig. 93) is taken through the malleoli; section B (fig. 94) is more anterior and runs through the sustentaculum tali and the peroneal tubercle.

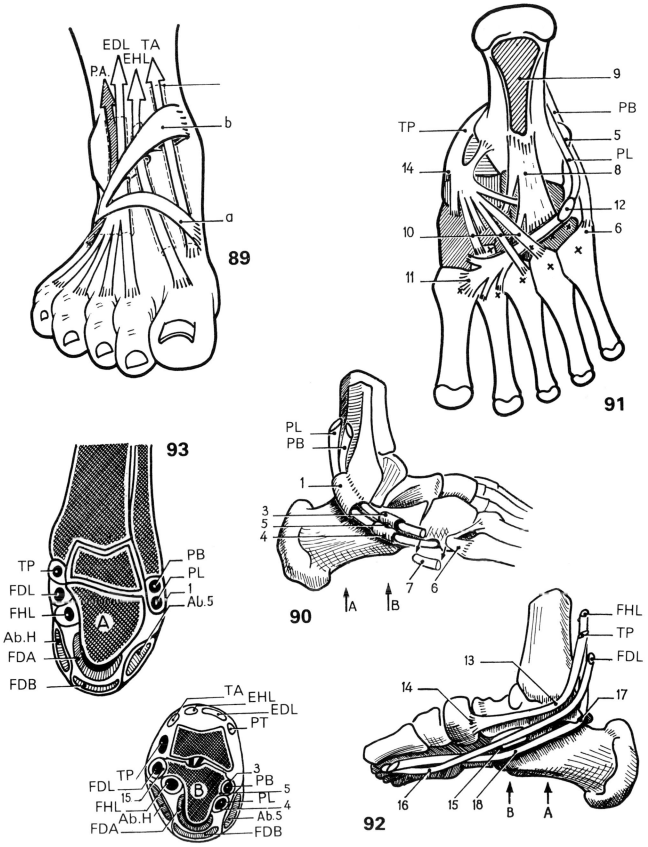

THE FLEXOR MUSCLES OF THE ANKLE

The foot as a whole and its posterior half are mobilized by the flexors and extensors of the knee acting about the axes of the articular complex of the posterior tarsus, as demonstrated previously (fig. 95). It seems to us best to give up Ombredanne's original schema (fig. 86) with the axes XX' and ZZ' perpendicular to each other; it does not fit the facts. By definition, the axes XX' and UU' of the 'heterokinetic universal joint' are not perpendicular to each other and this introduces a directional bias for the movements, a bias reinforced by the unequal distribution of the muscles. These axes give rise to four quadrants, in which are distributed *ten muscles* and thirteen tendons.

All the muscles **lying in front of the transverse axis XX' are flexors** of the ankle but these can be further subdivided into two groups according to their relationship to the long axis ZZ':

The two muscles lying medial to this axis, i.e. the extensor hallucis longus (EHL) and the tibialis anterior (TA) also produce *abduction* and *supination* simultaneously. The tibialis anterior, lying farther away from the axis ZZ', is more powerful as an adductor and supinator.

The two muscles lying lateral to the axis ZZ', i.e. the extensor digitorum longus (EDL) and the peroneus tertius (PT) are at the same time *abductors* and *pronators*. For the same reason, the peroneus is a more powerful abductor and pronator than the extensor digitorum.

Therefore to achieve pure flexion of the ankle, without any associated adduction and supination or abduction and pronation, these two muscle groups must contract simultaneously and in balanced fashion. Thus they are **antagonists and synergists**.

Of the four flexors of the ankle two are inserted directly into the tarsal or metatarsal bones:

the tibialis anterior (fig. 97) is inserted into the medial cuneiform and the first metatarsal;

the peroneus tertius (fig. 98), which is present in only 90 per cent. of cases is inserted into the dorsum of the base of the fifth metatarsal.

Their action on the foot is thus direct and requires no assistance from other muscles.

This is not the case with the other two flexors of the ankle: the extensor digitorum longus (EDL) and the extensor hallucis longus (EHL) which act on the foot via the toes. Thus if the toes are stabilised in the straight position or in flexion (fig. 98) by the interossei (Ix), the extensor digitorum longus flexes the ankle, but, if the interossei are paralysed ankle flexion is then accompanied by a claw-like deformity of the toes. Likewise (fig. 97) stabilisation of the big toe by the flexor hallucis longus and the abductor hallucis allows the extensor hallucis longus to flex the ankle; if these muscles are paralysed ankle flexion will be accompanied by a 'claw toe' (fig. 100).

When the muscles of the anterior compartment of the leg (fig. 99) are paralysed or insufficient, as occurs relatively commonly, the tips of the toes cannot be elevated: this is called 'pes equinus' (equus = horse, which walks on tiptoe). Thus, during walking, the patient must lift the whole leg fairly high so as to clear the ground. In certain cases, the extensor digitorum longus retains some of its power so that the dropped foot is also everted: this is valgus equinus (fig. 101).

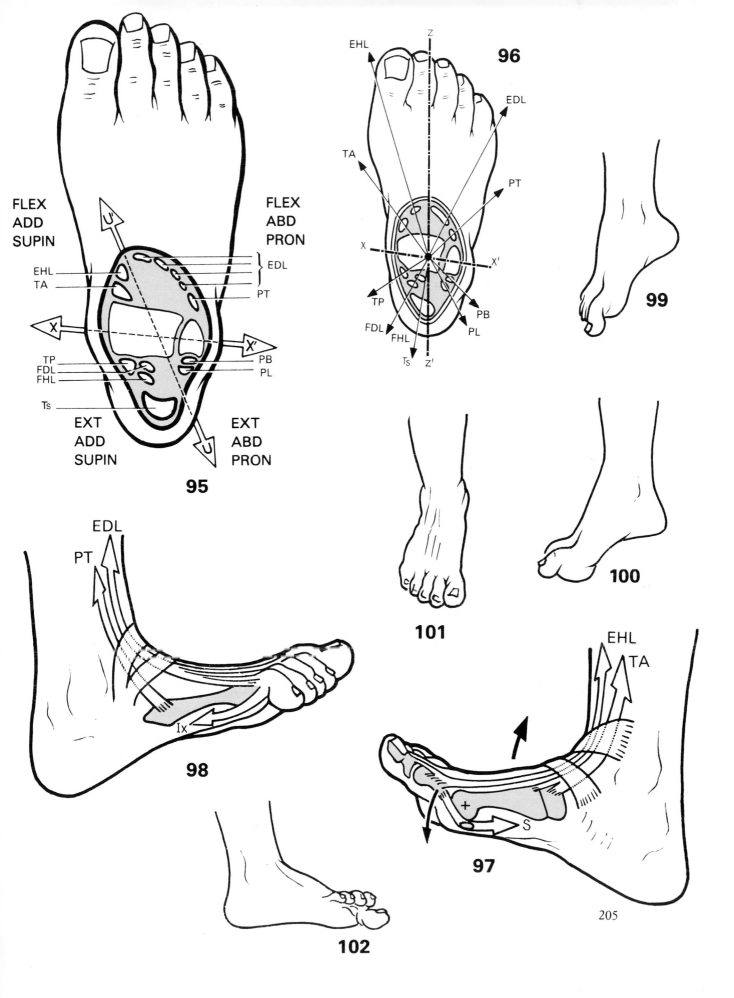

95

FLEX ADD SUPIN

FLEX ABD PRON

EHL
TA
EDL
PT

TP
FDL
FHL
PB
PL

Ts

EXT ADD SUPIN

EXT ABD PRON

96

Z

EHL
EDL
TA
PT
X
X'
TP
PB
FDL
PL
FHL
Ts
Z'

99

98

EDL
PT
Ix

101

100

102

97

EHL
TA
+
S

205

THE TRICEPS SURAE

All the extensors of the ankle lie *posterior to the axis XX′ of flexion and extension* (fig. 96). Theoretically there are six extensors of the ankle (discounting the plantaris which is negligible). In practice, however, only the triceps surae (gastrocnemius and soleus) are efficient extensors, constituting together one of the most powerful muscles of the body after the gluteus maximus and the quadriceps femoris. On the other hand, its axial position relative to ZZ′ makes it primarily an extensor.

This muscle group consists of **three muscle bellies** (fig. 103) which are inserted by a common tendon—*the Achilles tendon* (1)—into the posterior aspect of the calcaneus (p. 208). Of these three muscle bellies only one is monoarticular, the **soleus** (2), which arises from the tibia, the fibula and a fibrous band stretching between these two bones (3). It is deeply situated—seen here through the gastrocnemius—and surfaces only at the distal end on either side of the Achilles tendon. The other two muscle bellies—the **gastrocnemius**—are biarticular. **The lateral head** (3) arises from an impression above the lateral femoral condyle and from the 'condylar plate' which occasionally contains a sesamoid bone. The **medial head** (5) takes origin from the popliteal surface of the femur above the medial condyle and from the medial 'condylar plate'. These two muscle bellies converge inferiorly towards the midline and form the lower V of the diamond-shaped **popliteal fossa** (10). On either side they are flanked by the hamstring muscles which diverge proximally to form the upper V of the popliteal fossa; laterally by the biceps (6), medially by the sartorius, gracilis and semitendinosus (7). Between the gastrocnemius and the hamstrings *intervene two synovial bursae*: one bursa between the semitendinosus and the medial head of gastrocnemius (8), always present; and the other bursa (9) between the biceps and the lateral head, occasionally present. These bursae can give rise to popliteal cysts. The gastrocnemius and the soleus terminate in a complex aponeurosis which gives rise to the true Achilles tendon.

These three muscles **show unequal degrees of shortening** (fig. 104): the soleus (Cs) 44 mm. the gastrocnemius (Cg) 39 mm. This explains why the efficiency of the biarticular gastrocnemius *depends closely on the degree of flexion of the knee* (fig. 105): as the knee is fully flexed or fully extended the displacement of the origin of the muscle produces a relative lengthening or shortening of the muscle (e), which is equal to or exceeds its length of contraction. Thus when the knee is extended (fig. 106) the gastrocnemius passively stretched works at its best advantage and this allows some of the power of the quadriceps to be transferred to the ankle. On the other hand, when the knee is flexed (fig. 108) the gastrocnemius is maximally slackened (e is greater than Cg) and loses all its efficiency. Thus only *the soleus is active* but its power would be inadequate in walking, riding or jumping unless knee extension was an essential part of the process. Note that the gastrocnemius is not a knee flexor in spite of its position.

Any movement leading to simultaneous extension of ankle and knee, i.e. climbing (fig. 107) or running (figs. 109 and 110) promotes the action of the gastrocnemius. **The triceps surae achieves maximal efficiency** when, starting from the position of flexed ankle-extended knee, it contracts to extend the ankle (fig. 110) and to provide the *propulsive force in the last phase of the step*.

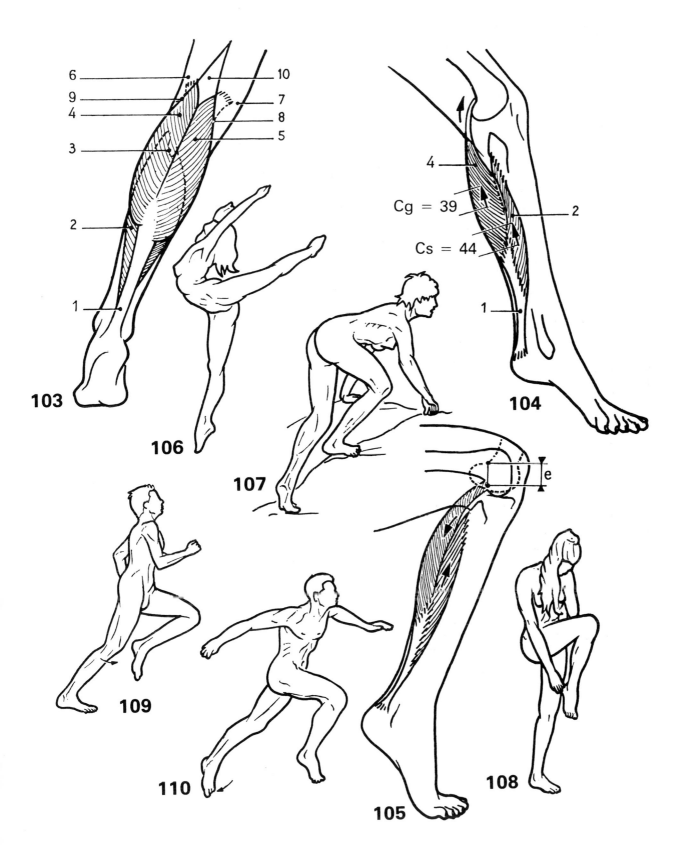

103

104

$Cg = 39$

$Cs = 44$

e

106

107

109

110

108

105

207

THE TRICEPS SURAE—(Continued)

The triceps surae has a very complex aponeurotic system (fig. 111: anterior view with tibia removed), comprising tendons of origin and tendons of insertion, which form the Achilles tendon distally.

There are three tendons of origin:

the two tendons of the *medial* (1) *and lateral* (2) *heads of the gastrocnemius*, arising from the supracondylar femoral shaft, form the superior border of the aponeurotic complex;

the *thick tendinous sheet of the soleus* (3) arises from the tibia and the fibula and its inferior portion is shaped like a horseshoe with a medial (4) and a lateral (5) horn.

There are two tendons of insertion:

a *thick common terminal sheet* (6), parallel to the soleus and giving rise to the Achilles tendon before its insertion into the calcaneus;

a *sagittal sheet* (7), perpendicular to the former and attached to it anteriorly. It thins out as it ascends up the soleus between the two horns of the horseshoe.

In the postero-anterior direction there are thus three successive aponeurotic planes: that of the gastrocnemius, then that of the common terminal sheet and that of the soleal tendons of origin, which are overridden by the sagittal sheet.

The **muscular fibres of the triceps surae** are arranged with respect to the aponeurotic complex as follows (fig. 112):

the *fibres of the medial (Gm) and of the lateral (Gl) heads of the gastrocnemius* arise from the anterior aspects of their tendons of origin, arch over the femoral condyles and run inferiorly and anteriorly towards the axis of the leg before *inserting into the common terminal sheet.*

The **muscular fibres of the soleus** are arranged in two planes:

the *posterior* (SP) with its fibres inserting into the anterior aspect of the terminal sheet and to a lesser degree into the medial and lateral aspects of the sagittal sheet;

the **anterior** with its medial fibres (ASM) inserting into the medial aspect of the sagittal sheet and its lateral fibres (ASL) inserting into the lateral aspect of the sagittal sheet.

This schematic digram also suggests the spiral arrangement of the Achilles tendon, which is responsible for its elasticity.

The force of the Achilles tendon is applied to the posterior surface of the calcaneus (fig. 113) along a line which forms a *wide angle* with its lever arm AO. When this force is resolved into two vectors, it is found that the effective vector T_1, i.e. perpendicular to the lever arm, is much greater than the centripetal vector t_2. Therefore *the muscle works at a high mechanical advantage.*

The effective component t_1 is always greater than t_2 whatever the degree of flexion or extension of the ankle. This is due to the **mode of insertion** of the tendon (fig. 114): it is inserted into the lower part of the posterior surface of the calcaneus (K) while it is separated from the upper part by a bursa. The muscular pull therefore is applied not at the point of insertion (K) but at the point of contact (A) of the tendon with the posterior surface of the bone. With the ankle flexed (a, fig. 114) this point A lies relatively far up on the posterior surface of the calcaneus. With the ankle extended (b, fig. 114) the tendon moves away from the bone and its point of contact A′ now lies farther down but *the direction of the lever arm A′O still remains clearly horizontal, forming a constant angle with the line of the tendon.* This mode of insertion of the Achilles tendon allows the tendon to 'uncoil' on the pulley segment formed by the posterior surface of the calcaneus and this **increases its efficiency during ankle extension**; it resembles the insertion of the triceps brachii into the olecranon process (see Vol. 1).

When the triceps surae contracts maximally (fig. 115), the movement of extension is associated with a **movement of adduction and supination** so that the sole of the foot faces posteriorly and medially (arrow). This is due to the fact that the **triceps surae acts on the ankle joint through the subtalar joint** (fig. 116). It mobilises these joints in succession (fig. 117): first of all it extends the ankle through 30° around the transverse axis XX′; then acting at the subtalar joint it tilts the calcaneus about the axis of Henke (mn) so that the foot is adducted by 13° and supinated by 12° (Biesalski and Mayer, 1916).

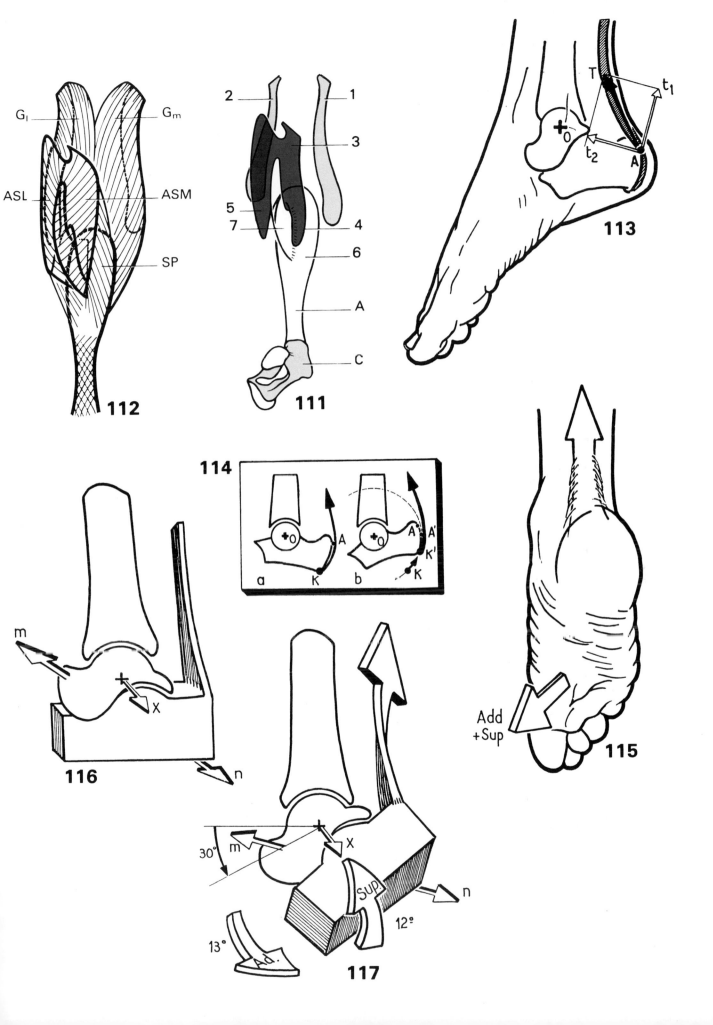

112

G_l · · · G_m

ASL · · · ASM

· · · SP

111

2 · · · 1

· · · 3

5 · · ·

7 · · · 4

· · · 6

· · · A

· · · C

113

T

t_1

+O

t_2

A

114

+O A

a K

+O A'' A'

K'

b K

115

Add +Sup

116

m

+

X

n

117

30°

m

X

Sup.

13°

12°

n

THE OTHER EXTENSOR MUSCLES OF THE ANKLE

All the muscles running posterior to the transverse axis XX′ of flexion and extension (fig. 118) are extensors of the ankle. In addition to the triceps surae (T), **five other muscles** extend the ankle: the plantaris (not described here) is so weak as to be negligible and it is only important in providing a ready tendon for transplantation; unfortunately it is not always present.

Laterally (fig. 119), the peroneus brevis (PB) and the peroneus longus (PL), lying lateral to the long axis zz′ of the joint (fig. 95) simultaneously produce *abduction and pronation* (p. 212).

Medially (fig. 120), the tibialis posterior (TP), the flexor digitorum longus (FDL) and the flexor hallucis longus (FHL) lie medial to the axis zz′ (fig. 95) and so simultaneously produce *adduction* and *supination* (p. 214).

Pure extension can result only from balanced action of these lateral and medial muscles i.e. **synergists and antagonists**.

However, the extensor action of these muscles which can be called **accessory extensors**, is relatively slight compared with that of the triceps surae (fig. 121). In effect, the power of the triceps surae is equivalent to 65 kg. weight while the total power of these accessory extensors (f) is equivalent to 0·5 kg. weight, i.e. *one fourteenth of the total power available for extension*. The power of a muscle is proportional to its cross-sectional area and its length of contraction and so can be represented diagrammatically by a volume whose base is its cross-sectional area and whose height is its length of contraction. The soleus (sol), with cross-sectional area 20 cm^2 and contraction length 44 mm. is less powerful (880) than the gastrocnemius (897) with cross-sectional area 23 cm^2 and contraction length 39 mm. On the other hand, the power of the peroneal muscles (striped cube) represents *one half* of the total power of the accessory extensors. The peroneus longus is itself in turn twice as powerful as the peroneus brevis.

After rupture of the Achilles tendon, the accessory extensor muscles can actively extend the ankle when the foot is free and unsupported. But only the triceps surae can allow one to stand on tiptoe and loss of this movement is diagnostic of rupture of this tendon.

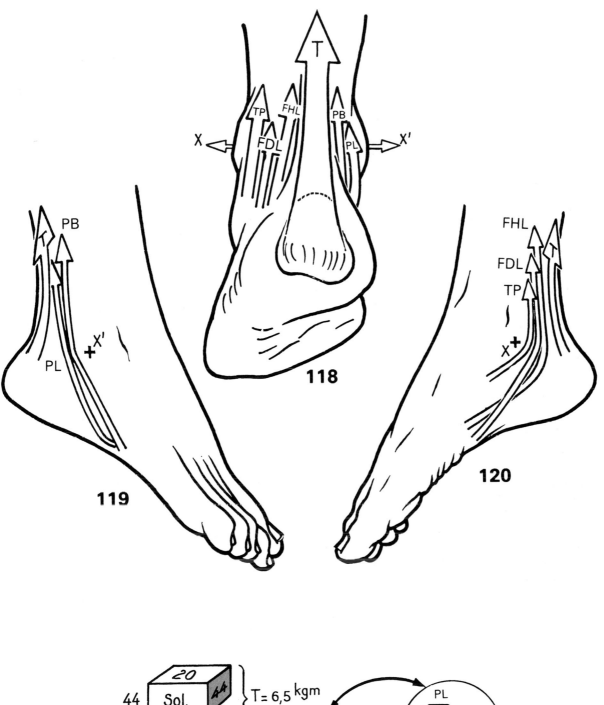

118

119

120

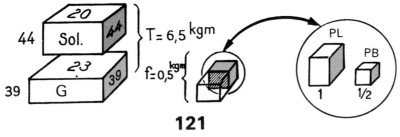

121

THE ABDUCTOR-PRONATOR MUSCLES: THE PERONEI

These muscles run posterior to the transverse axis XX' and lateral to Henke's axis UU' and so produce simultaneously (fig. 122):

extension (arrow 1);

abduction (arrow 2) so that the axis ZZ' is displaced laterally;

pronation (arrow 3) so that the sole of the foot faces laterally.

The **peroneus brevis** (PB), inserted (fig. 123) into the lateral tubercle of the base of the fifth metatarsal is primarily an abductor of the foot: according to Duchenne de Boulogne it is in fact the only pure abductor (see also fig. 90). Certainly, it is a more efficient abductor than the peroneus longus. It also produces (fig. 124) pronation of the anterior half of the foot (arrow 3) by lifting (arrow a) the lateral metatarsals: in this action it receives assistance from the peroneus tertius (PT) and the extensor digitorum longus (not shown here), which are also abductor-pronators of the foot while simultaneously flexing the ankle. Therefore pure abduction-pronation, results from the *synergistic-antagonistic action* of the peronei brevis and longus on the one hand and of the peroneus brevis and the extensor digitorum longus on the other.

The **peroneus longus** (PL) (figs. 123 and 125) plays a fundamental part both in the movements of the foot and in the statics and dynamics of the plantar arches:

1. It is an *abductor* like the peroneus brevis and contracture of the muscle causes the foot to be pulled laterally (fig. 127) while the medial malleolus sticks out more prominently.

2. It produces *extension* directly and especially indirectly:

directly (figs. 124 and 125), by lowering (arrow 6) the head of the first metatarsal;

indirectly, by pulling the first metatarsal laterally (arrow 5, fig. 125) so that the medial and lateral metatarsals form one solid piece, as it were. Now (fig. 126) the triceps surae, as an extensor, acts directly on only the lateral metatarsals (shown diagrammatically as a single beam): thus by 'coupling' the medial with the lateral metatarsals the peroneus longus allows the pull of the triceps to act on all the metatarsals at one time. This is confirmed by instances of paralysis of the peroneus longus where only the lateral arch is extended so that the foot is in fact supinated. **Pure extension of the foot** is therefore the result of the *synergistic-antagonistic* contraction of the triceps surae and the peroneus longus: synergistic in extension, antagonistic in rotation.

3. It is in effect a *pronator* muscle (fig. 124) as it lowers (arrow b) the head of the first metatarsal when the foot is clear of the ground. Pronation (arrow 3) results from elevation of the lateral arch (a) along with lowering of the medial arch (b).

It will become apparent later (p. 224) how the peroneus longus accentuates the curvature of the three arches of the foot and constitutes their main muscular support.

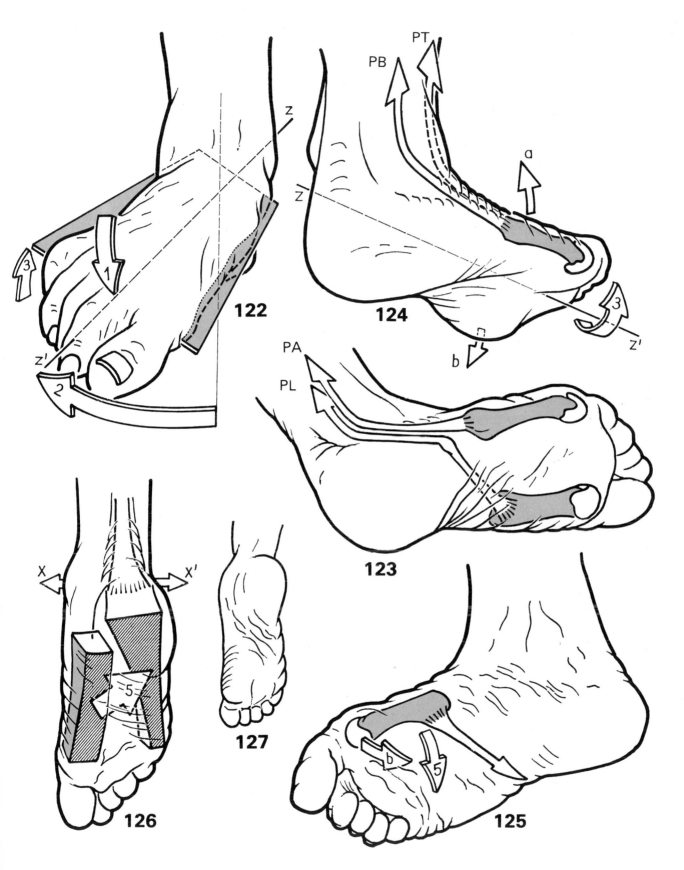

122

124

123

126

127

125

213

THE ADDUCTOR-SUPINATOR MUSCLES: THE TIBIALIS MUSCLES

The three muscles, lying posterior to the medial malleolus, run posterior to the axis XX' and medial to the axis UU' (fig. 95) and so produce simultaneously (fig. 128):

extension (arrow 1);

adduction (arrow 2), so that the axis ZZ' is displaced medially;

supination (arrow 3) so that the sole of the foot faces medially.

The **tibialis posterior** (TP), the most important of these three muscles, is inserted (fig. 129) into the tubercle of the navicular bone (shaded). As it crosses the ankle and the subtalar and transverse tarsal joints it acts simultaneously on all three:

By pulling the navicular medially (fig. 130) it is a **very powerful adductor** (according to Duchenne de Boulogne it is more of an adductor than supinator). Thus it is a *direct antagonist of the peroneus brevis* (PB), which draws the anterior part of the foot laterally (fig. 131) by acting on the fifth metatarsal.

As a result of its plantar attachments to the tarsal and metatarsal bones (fig. 91) it produces **supination** and plays a vital role in supporting and orientating the plantar arches (p. 224). Congenital absence of these plantar attachments has been blamed as one of the causes of the pes planus valgus. The total range of supination is 52° with 34° occurring at the talocalcanean joint and 18° at the transverse tarsal joint (Biesalski and Mayer).

It is an extensor (fig. 132) not only of the ankle (arrow a) but also of the transverse tarsal joint by lowering the navicular (arrow b): the ankle movement is continued by the movement of the anterior half of the foot (p. 153, fig. 5).

During extension and adduction, the tibialis posterior is helped by the flexor hallucis longus and by the flexor digitorum longus.

The tibialis anterior and the extensor hallucis longus (fig. 132) run *anterior* to the transverse axis XX' and medial to Henke's axis (fig. 95) and thus are at once *flexors, adductors* and *supinators* of the ankle.

The tibialis anterior (TA) and the extensor hallucis longus (EHL) pass (fig. 133) *anterior to* the transverse axis xx' and medial to Henke's axis UU' (fig. 95): they therefore produce simultaneously *flexion* of the ankle and *adduction* and *supination* of the foot.

The **tibialis anterior** (fig. 128) is more efficient as a supinator than an adductor. It acts by elevating all the structures of the medial arch (fig. 132):

It lifts the base of the first metatarsal on the medial cuneiform (arrow c) so that the metatarsal head is also elevated.

It lifts the medial cuneiform over the navicular (arrow d) and the navicular over the talus (arrow e) before flexing the ankle (arrow f).

It flattens the medial arch by producing supination of the foot and so is *the direct antagonist of the peroneus longus.*

It has a less powerful action as an adductor than the tibialis posterior.

It flexes the ankle and, in conjunction with its *synergist-antagonist* i.e. the tibialis posterior, it produces pure adduction and supination without flexion or extension.

Contracture of the tibialis anterior causes a pes talovarus with flexion deformity of the toes (fig. 134), especially of the big toe.

The **extensor hallucis longus** (fig. 133) is less powerful than the tibialis anterior in producing adduction and supination. It can replace the latter as a flexor of the ankle but it often produces 'clawing' of the big toe.

The power of the supinators (2·82 kg. weight) exceeds that of the pronators (1·16 kg. weight): in the absence of any support the foot spontaneously assumes a position in supination. This imbalance compensates beforehand for the natural tendency of the foot to be pronated (p. 226) when it supports the weight of the body on the ground.

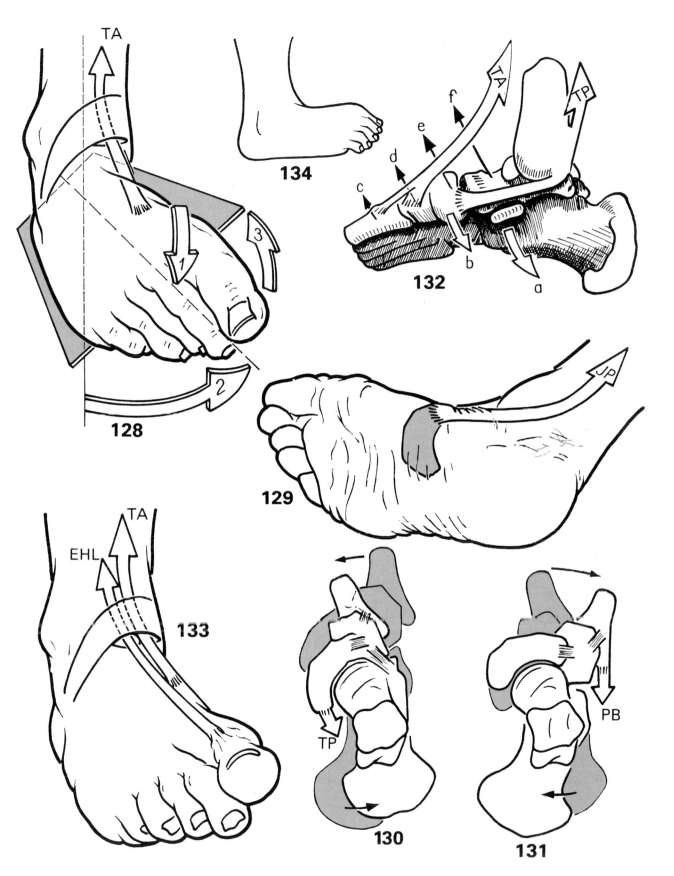

128

134

132

129

133

130

131

The Plantar Vault

The plantar vault is an **architectural structure** which blends all the elements of the foot—joints, ligaments and muscles—into a unified system. Thanks to its changes of curvature and its elasticity, the vault can adapt itself to unevenness of the ground and can transmit to the ground the forces exerted by the weight of the body and its movements. This it achieves with the best mechanical advantage under the most varied conditions. The plantar vault acts as a **shock-absorber** essential for the flexibility of the gait. Any pathological conditions, which exaggerate or flatten its curvatures, interfere seriously with the support of the body on the ground and necessarily with running, walking and the maintenance of the erect posture.

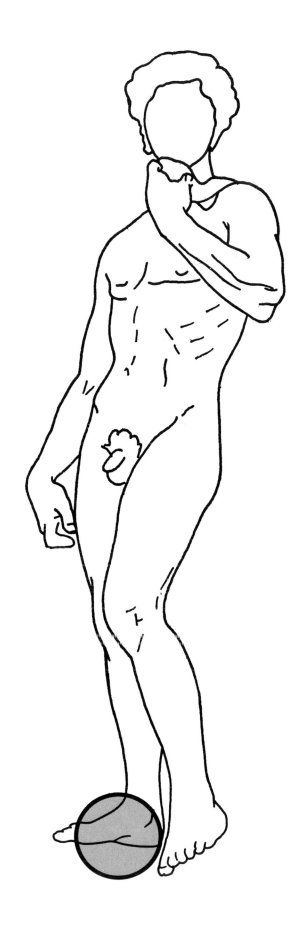

217

THE MEDIAL ARCH

Between its anterior (A) and posterior (C) supports the medial arch (fig. 7) comprises **five bones** which are as follows anteroposteriorly:

the *first metatarsal* (M_1) touches the ground only by its head (A);

the *medial cuneiform* (C_m), completely clear of the ground;

the *navicular* (nav.), which is the keystone of the arch (striped) and lies 15 to 18 cm. above the ground;

the *talus* (Tal), which receives all the forces transmitted by the leg and transmits them to the vault (fig. 34);

the *calcaneus* (Calc.) which is in contact with the ground only at its posterior extremity.

The transmission of the mechanical forces is reflected (fig. 8) in **the direction of the bony trabeculae:**

The trabeculae arising from the cortex of the anterior surface of the tibia run obliquely inferiorly and posteriorly through the posterior buttress of the arch. They traverse the body of the talus and fan out in the calcaneus to reach the posterior support of the arch.

The trabeculae arising from the cortex of the posterior surface of the tibia run obliquely inferiorly and anteriorly and traverse the neck and head of the talus, the navicular and the anterior buttress, i.e. the medial cuneiform and the metatarsal.

The medial arch maintains its concavity only *with the help of ligaments and muscles* (fig. 7).

Many **plantar ligaments** unite these five bones: cuneometatarsal, cuneonavicular, but especially the *plantar calcaneonavicular ligament* (1) and the *talocalcanean ligament* (2). These resist violent but short-lasting stresses whereas the muscles cope with sustained strains.

The **muscles** join two points, which lie at varying distances along the arch, and span either the whole of the arch or part of it. They therefore act as **tighteners** of the various arches.

The **tibialis posterior** (TP) spans part of the medial arch (fig. 10) near its dome but it plays a vital part. In fact (fig. 9) it pulls back the navicular inferiorly and posteriorly under the head of the talus (circle with circumference in broken line). This relatively trivial shortening of the muscle (e) is associated with a change in direction of the navicular so that the anterior buttress of the arch is lowered. Moreover, its plantar attachments (3, fig. 7) blend with the plantar ligaments and act on the three middle metatarsals.

The **peroneus longus** (PL) also acts on the medial arch and accentuates its curvature (fig. 11) by flexing M_1 on the medial cuneiform and the latter on the navicular (fig. 9); (see also p. 224 for its action on the transverse arch).

The **flexor hallucis longus** (FHL) spans most of the medial arch (fig. 12) and so has a powerful influence on its curvature; in this action it is assisted by the **flexor digitorum longus** (FDL) which crosses it from below (fig. 13). The flexor hallucis longus also acts to stabilise the talus and the calcaneus: as it runs between the two tubercles of the talus it prevents the talus (r) from receding (fig. 14) when pushed back by the navicular (white arrow): the talocalcanean interosseous ligament (2) is first stretched and *the talus is restored to its original position anteriorly* by the tendon which propels it forward just as a bowstring propels an arrow. As it runs below the sustentaculum tali (fig. 15) the flexor hallucis longus (by a similar mechanism) re-elevates the anterior half of the calcaneus which receives the vertical force transmitted by the head of the talus (white arrow).

The **abductor hallucis longus** (Ab. HL.) spans the whole medial arch (fig. 16). It is therefore a particularly efficient tightener: it accentuates the curvature of the arch by approximating its two ends.

On the other hand (fig. 17) the two muscles inserted into the convexity of the arch, i.e. the extensor hallucis longus (EHL)—under certain conditions—and the tibialis anterior (TA) reduce its curvature and flatten the arch.

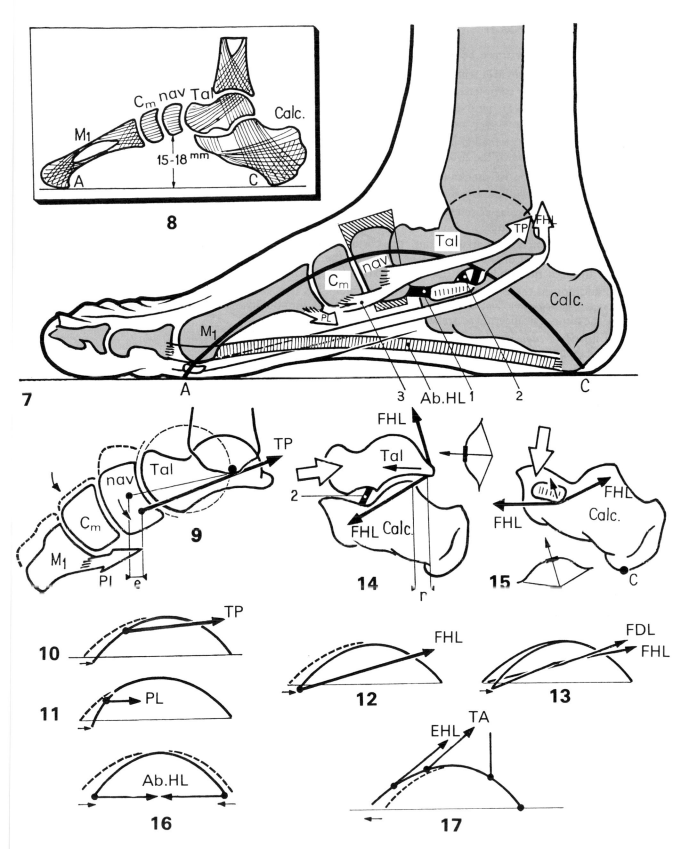

THE ANTERIOR ARCH AND THE TRANSVERSE CURVATURE OF THE FOOT

The anterior arch (fig. 27, section I) runs from **the head of the first metatarsal (A)**, **which rests on two sesamoid bones** and is 6 mm. above the ground, to **the head of the fifth metatarsal (B)**, which also lies 6 mm. above the ground. It traverses the heads of the intervening metatarsals. The **head of the second metatarsal**, which is the highest above the ground (9 mm.), is the *keystone* of the arch. The head of the third (8·5 mm.) and of the fourth (7 mm.) metatarsals occupy intermediate positions.

The arch is relatively flat and rests on the ground via the soft tissues, often called the 'anterior heel' of the foot. It is spanned on its plantar surface by the relatively weak intermetatarsal ligaments and by only one muscle—the **transverse head of the adductor hallucis (Ad. H)**. Some fibres of the adductor span the whole length of the arch while others span only part of it running from the head of the first metatarsal, to each of the other metatarsal heads. This muscle is relatively weak and gives way very easily. The arch is often flattened—flat forefoot—or even reversed—the convex forefoot—so that callosities are formed on the lowered metatarsal heads (p. 240).

The *anterior arch is the point of culmination of the five metatarsal rays of the foot.* The first ray (fig. 29) is the highest and forms (Fick) an angle of 18° to 25° with the ground. This angle between the metatarsal and ground decreases regularly, being 15° for the second ray (fig. 30), 10° of the third (fig. 31), 8° for the fourth (fig. 32) and only 5° for the fifth (fig. 33), which is nearly parallel to the ground.

The transverse arch of the foot involves the whole length of the foot. **At the level of the cuneiforms** (fig. 27, section II) it comprises only four bones and rests on the ground only at its lateral extremity, i.e. the cuboid (Cub). The medial cuneiform (C_m) is quite clear of the ground; the intermediate cuneiform (C_i) is the keystone of the arch (striped) and constitutes with the second metatarsal the axis of the foot, i.e. **the crest-tile of the vault**. This arc of a circle is subtended by the tendon of the peroneus longus (PL) which thus exerts a powerful action on the transverse curvature of the foot.

At the level of the navicular and the cuboid (fig. 27, section III) the transverse arch rests only on its lateral extremity, i.e. the cuboid (Cub). The navicular (nav) is slung above the ground and overhangs the medial surface of the cuboid. The curvature of this arch depends on the plantar expansions of the tibialis posterior (TP).

A plantar view of the left foot (assumed to be transparent) shows (fig. 28) how the **transverse arch** is maintained by three muscles successively anteroposteriorly:

the adductor hallucis (Ad. H) which runs transversely;

the peroneus longus (PL), the most important muscle in the dynamics of the foot, acts as a tightening device running obliquely anteriorly and medially: it acts **on the three arches of the foot**;

the plantar expansions of the tibialis posterior (TP), especially important in the statics of the foot, act as a tightener running obliquely anteriorly and laterally.

The **longitudinal curvature** of the foot as a whole depends on:

medially, the *abductor hallucis* (Ab. H) and the flexor hallucis longus (not shown);

laterally, the *abductor digiti minimi* (Ab. 5).

Between these two extreme tighteners the flexor digitorum longus, the flexor digitorum accessorius (not shown) and the flexor digitorum brevis (FDB) maintain the curvature of the three intermediate rays as well as that of the fifth ray.

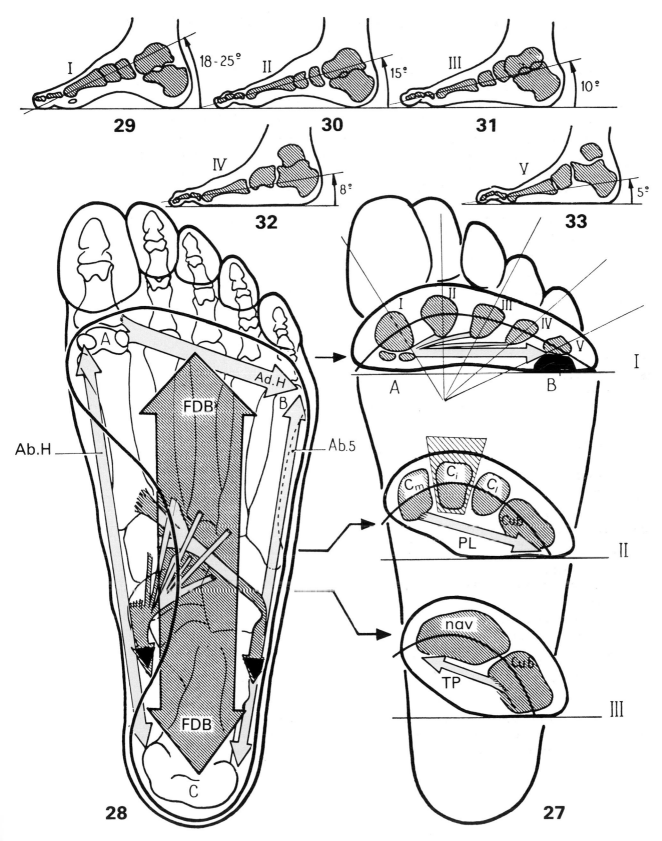

29   30   31

32   33

28   27

225

THE DISTRIBUTION OF STRESSES AND THE STATIC DISTORTIONS OF THE PLANTAR VAULT

The weight of the body, transmitted by the lower limb, is applied through the ankle to the posterior part of the foot (fig. 34) at the level of the trochlear surface of the talus. From there the forces are distributed in three directions towards the supports of the vault:

towars the anterior and medial support (A), via the neck of the talus and the anterior buttress of the medial arch;

towards the anterior and lateral support (B), via the head of the talus, the sustentaculum tali of the calcaneus and the anterior buttress of the lateral arch;

towards the posterior support (C) via the body of the talus, the subtalar joint, and the body of the calcaneus (the bony trabeculae underlying the superior articular surface) i.e. through the common posterior buttress of the medial and lateral arches.

The relative distribution of these forces to each support is easily remembered (fig. 35) as follows: if 6 kg. weight is applied, 1 kg. is applied to the anterolateral support (B), 2 kg. to the anteromedial support (A) and 3 kg. to the posterior support (C) (Morton, 1935). When the body is in the erect position, straight and stationary, the heel bears the brunt of the stress, i.e. about half of the body weight. This explains why, when this force is applied through a fine stiletto heel, plastic materials on the floor are easily 'punched in'.

Under the body weight each arch of the foot is flattened and lengthened.

The medial arch (fig. 36): the posterior tubercles of the calcaneum which are 7 to 10 mm. above the ground, are lowered by 1·5 mm. and the sustentaculum tali of the calcaneus by 4 mm.; the talus recedes on the calcaneus; the navicular rises on the head of the talus while moving nearer to the ground; the cuneonavicular and the cuneometatarsal joints gape open inferiorly; the angle between the first metatarsal and the ground is reduced; the heel recedes and the sesamoid bones move a little anteriorly.

The lateral arch (fig. 37): similar vertical displacements of the calcaneus; the cuboid is lowered by 4 mm., the lateral tubercle of the fifth metatarsal by 3·5 mm.; the calcaneocuboid and cubometatarsal joints gape open inferiorly; the heel recedes and the head of the fifth metatarsal moves forward slightly.

The anterior arch (fig. 38): the arch is flattened and splayed out on either side of the second metatarsal. The distance between the first and second metatarsals increases by 5 mm., that between the second and third by 2 mm., that between the third and the fourth by 4 mm. and that between the fourth and the fifth by 1·5 mm. Therefore the *forefoot is widened* by 12·5 mm. when bearing the weight of the body.

The transverse curvature is also reduced at the level of the cuneiforms (fig. 39) and at the level of the navicular (fig. 40), while these two transverse arches tend to be tilted laterally by an angle x, which is proportional to the degree of flattening of the medial arch.

In addition (fig. 41) the head of the talus is displaced medially by 2 to 6 mm. and the lateral tubercle of the calcaneus by 2 to 4 mm. This leads to *twisting of the foot at the transverse tarsal joint*: the axis of the hindfoot is displaced medially while that of the forefoot moves laterally forming an angle of y with the former. The hindfoot turns into adduction-pronation (arrow 1) and slight extension while the forefoot undergoes a *relative* movement of flexion-abduction-supination (arrow 2). This phenomenon is particularly conspicuous in the *pes planus valgus* (p. 238).

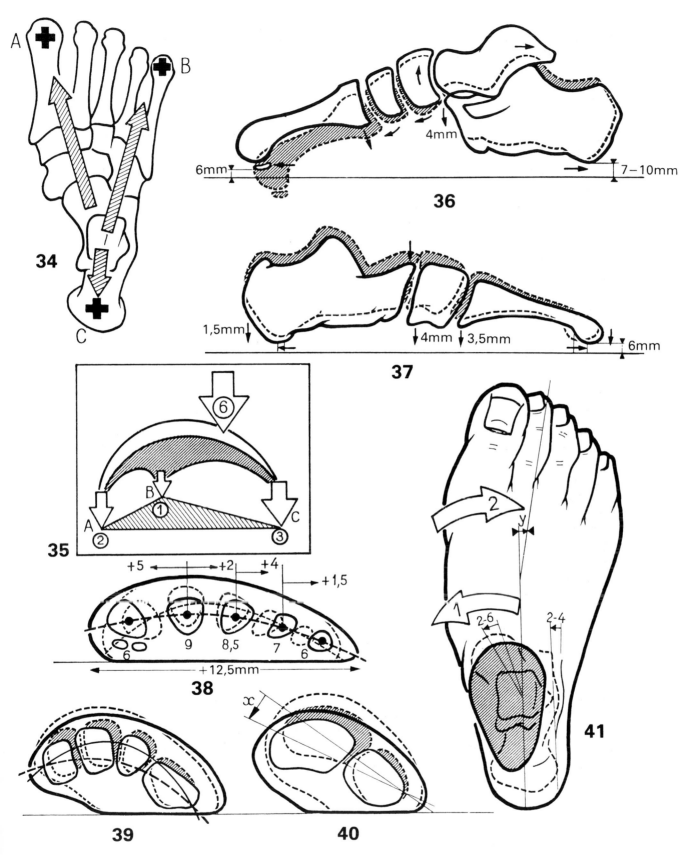

34

36

6mm
4mm
7–10mm

37

1,5mm
4mm 3,5mm
6mm

35

6

B
A 2
1
C 3

38

+5 +2 +4
+1,5
9 8,5 7 6
6
+12,5mm

39

40

x

41

2
1
2-6
2-4
y

227

THE ARCHITECTURAL EQUILIBRIUM OF THE FOOT

The foot is a triangular structure (fig. 42) with:

an inferior side (A), i.e. the base or the plantar vault, subtended by the plantar muscles and ligaments;

an anterosuperior side (B), comprising the flexors of the ankle and the extensors of the toes;

a posterior side (C), comprising the extensors of the ankle and the flexors of the toes.

The normal shape of the plantar vault, which allows the foot to adapt correctly to the grounds, is the result of an equilibrium among the forces acting along these three sides of the triangle (fig. 43). These sides in vivo consist of a series of bones bound together at the ankle joint and the articular complex of the posterior tarsus.

Thus pes cavus, due to an exaggerated plantar vault, can result from shortening of the plantar ligaments, contracture of the plantar muscles and deficiency of the flexors of the ankle. Pes planus, due to flattening of the plantar vault, can result from insufficiency of the plantar ligaments or muscles and from hypertonicity of the anterior or posterior muscles of the foot.

This is yet another example of the concept of trilateral equilibrium, illustrated by the surfing board.

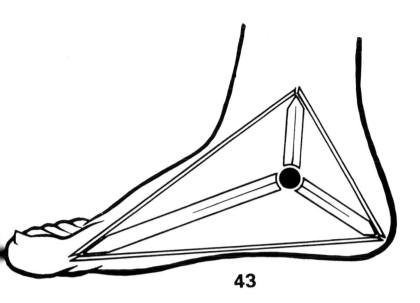

43

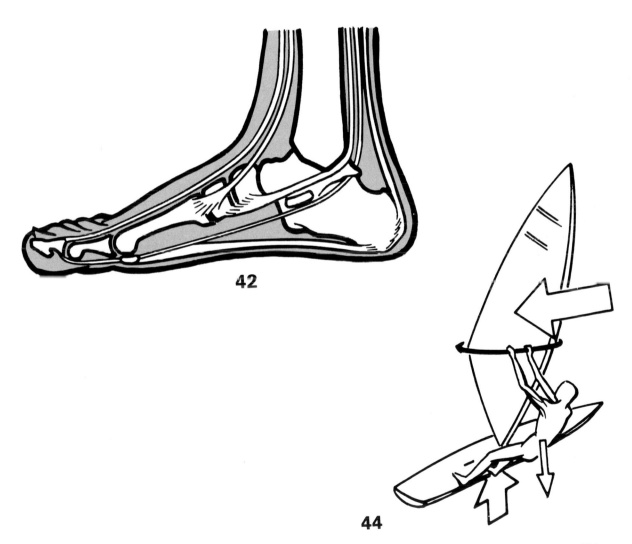

42

44

DYNAMIC CHANGES OF THE ARCHES OF THE FOOT DURING WALKING

During walking the **evolution of the step** subjects these arches to stresses and strains, which highlight the function of these arches as an *elastic shock-absorber*. The 'unwinding' of the step has **four phases**.

Phase I: Contact with the ground is established (fig. 45).

When the forward limb is about to 'land' the ankle is straight or slightly flexed (fig. 45) by the action of the ankle flexors (F). The foot touches the ground **at the heel**, i.e. at the posterior support of the plantar vault. Straight away, under the thrust of the leg (white arrow), the foot is flattened on the ground (arrow 1) while the ankle is passively extended.

Phase II: Maximum contact (fig. 46).

The sole of the foot rests on the ground over the whole of its bearing surface which constitutes *the footprint*. **The body, propelled by the other foot, passes first vertically over the supporting limb and then moves in front of it** (period of unilateral support). Thus the ankle changes passively from the position of extension to a new position of flexion (arrow 2). At the same time, the weight of the body (white arrow) is fully applied to the plantar vault which is flattened. This flattening of the vault is simultaneously checked by contraction of the plantar tighteners (P)—the first stage of shock absorption. As it flattens, the vault is lengthened a little: at the start of this movement the anterior support (A) moves anteriorly slightly but at the end, when the anterior support becomes more and more firmly fixed to the ground under the weight of the body, the posterior support C, i.e. the heel, recedes. The surface area of the footprint is maximal when the leg is vertically above the foot.

Phase III: First stage of active propulsion (fig. 47).

The weight of the body is shifted to the anterior part of the supporting foot and **contraction of the ankle extensors** (T), especially **the triceps surae, raises the heel** (arrow 3). While the ankle is thus actively extended the plantar vault as a whole rotates about its anterior support (A). The body is lifted and moves anteriorly: this is the first stage of propulsion and is especially important as it depends on powerful muscles. Meanwhile, the plantar vault, caught between the ground anteriorly, the muscular force posteriorly and the weight of the body centrally (lever of the second type), would be flattened if the plantar tighteners (P) did not intervene: this is the second stage of shock absorption which allows some of the force of the triceps to be stored for release at the end of the propulsive movement. On the other hand, it is at the moment when the body is supported on the anterior part of the foot that the anterior arch is flattened in its turn (fig. 48) and the anterior part of the foot is splayed out on the ground (fig. 49).

Phase IV: Second stage of active propulsion (fig. 50).

The force provided by the triceps surae is followed by a second propulsive force (arrow 4) supplied by contraction of the flexors of the toes (f), especially the flexor hallucis brevis, the adductor and the abductor hallucis and the flexor hallucis longus. The foot is now once more raised further anteriorly and is no longer supported by the anterior tarsal bones; it now rests entirely on the first three toes (fig. 51), especially the big toe—the final stage of support (A'). During this second propulsive movement the plantar vault resists flattening once more thanks to the plantar tighteners, comprising the flexors of the toes *inter alia*. It is at this stage that the energy stored by these tighteners is released. The foot then leaves the ground while the other starts a new step. Thus both feet are in contact with the ground for a very short time (period of bilateral support). In the next stage—i.e. of unilateral support—the vault of the foot which has just left the ground moves back to its original position.

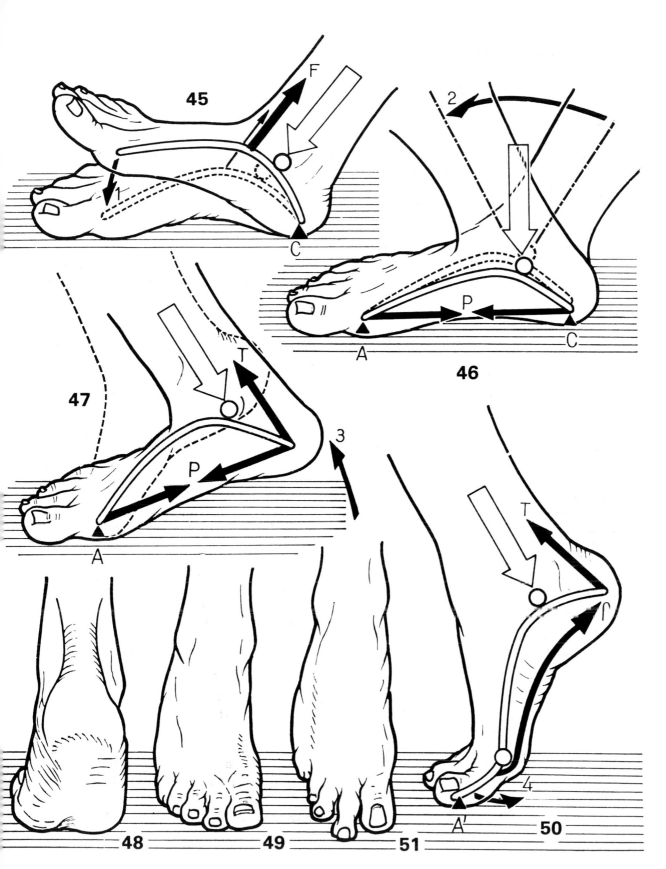

DYNAMIC CHANGES RELATED TO THE MEDIAL AND LATERAL INCLINATION OF THE LEG ON THE FOOT

So far we have studied the alterations occurring in the plantar vault during walking, i.e. following changes of the angle between leg and foot in *the sagittal plane*. During walking or running along a *curved track or uneven ground* it is essential that the leg should be able to change the angle it forms with the foot in **the frontal plane**, i.e. medial and lateral to the footprint. These side-to-side movements take place at the **subtalar and transverse tarsal joints** and lead to changes in the shape of the plantar vault. Note that the ankle is not involved: *the talus, gripped between the two malleoli, moves relative to the other tarsal bones.*

When the leg is inclined medially with respect to the foot (considered to be stationary) the following four changes take place (fig. 51):

1. *Lateral rotation of the leg on the foot* (arrow 1) which takes place only when the sole of the foot is firmly fixed on the ground. It is recognised clinically by the posterior movement of the lateral malleolus relative to its position when the foot, perpendicular to the leg, is in contact with the ground only along its medial border (fig. 52). This lateral rotation of the two malleoli leads to a lateral displacement of the talus, especially of its head lodged in the navicular.

2. *Abduction-supination of the hindfoot* (fig. 53). The abduction is due to an uncompensated component of lateral rotation. Supination results from medial displacement of the calcaneus which is obvious from the back (angle x) and when referred to a foot clear of the ground (fig. 54). This 'varus' movement of the calcaneus is associated with a change of the medial border of the Achilles tendon from straight to concave.

3. *Adduction-pronation of the forefoot* (fig. 51). When the anterior arch is applied to the ground the anterior part of the foot is displaced medially: its axis passing through the second metatarsal and the sagittal plane P passing through this axis are tilted medially through an angle m (P′ represents the final position of this plane and P its initial position), which is a measure of this movement of adduction. The anterior part of the foot is also pronated. But it is clear that **these movements of adduction and pronation are only relative to those of the hindfoot.** They occur at the transverse tarsal joint.

4. *'Hollowing' of the medial arch* (fig. 51). This increase in the curvature of the medial arch (arrow 2) is itself a consequence of the relative movements of the anterior and posterior parts of the foot. It is associated with elevation of the navicular relative to the ground: this elevation is at once passive (lateral displacement of the talar head) and active (contraction of the tibialis posterior). The overall change in the curvature of the plantar vault is seen in the change in its outline: the hollow of the foot deepens as in the case of a *pes cavus varus.*

When the leg is inclined laterally (fig. 55) four symmetrical changes occur:

1. *Medial rotation of the leg on the foot* (arrow 3): posterior displacement of the medial malleolus (cf. with fig. 52 where the foot only rests on its lateral margin); medial movement of the talus so that its head projects on the medial border of the foot.

2. *Adduction-pronation of the hindfoot* (fig. 57): adduction due to an uncompensated component of medial rotation; pronation with valgus (angle y) of the calcaneus (cf. fig. 58).

3. *Abduction-supination of the forefoot* (fig. 55): angle (n) of abduction between the two planes P and P′.

4. *Flattening of the medial arch* (arrow 4): the surface area of the footprint is increased, as in the *pes planus valgus.*

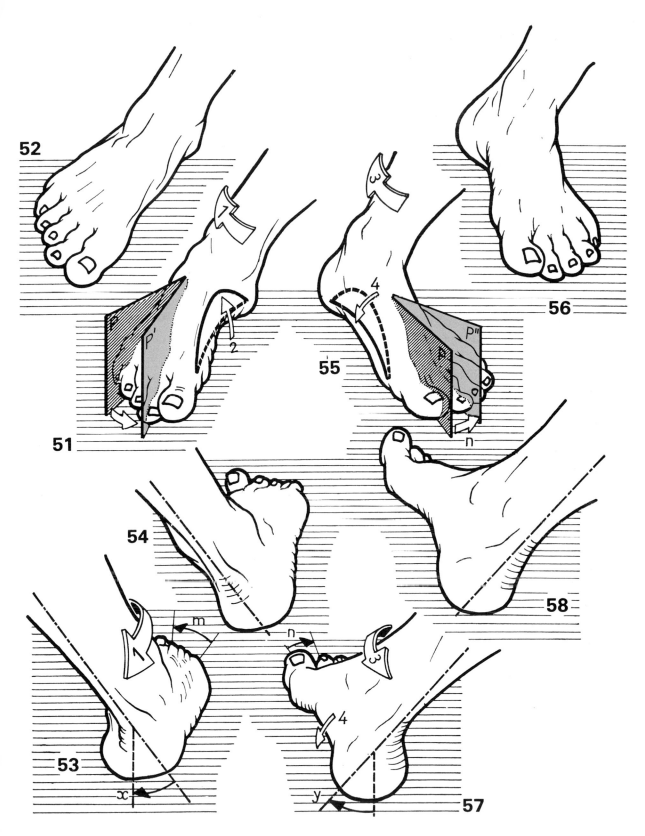

ADAPTATION OF THE PLANTAR VAULT TO THE GROUND

The town dweller always walks on even and firm ground with his feet protected by shoes. There is therefore little need for the arches of his feet to adapt to new terrains and the supporting muscles eventually atrophy: the flat foot is the price paid for progress and some anthropologists go so far as to forecast that man's feet will be reduced to mere stumps. This thesis is borne out by the fact that in man in contrast to the ape the toes are atrophied and the big toe can no longer be opposed.

This stage is still to come and even 'civilised' man can still walk barefoot on a beach or on the rocks. This return to the primitive state is highly beneficial to the plantar vault (*inter alia*), which thus retrieves its adaptive capabilities:

Adaptation to the uneven features of the ground, which the foot can grasp within the hollow of the vault (fig. 59).

Adaptation to slopes of the ground with respect to the feet: the bearing surface of the forefoot is more extensive *when the ground slopes laterally*, because of the decreasing lengths of the metatarsal bones mediolaterally (fig. 60):

when one *stands on a transverse slope* (fig. 61) the foot 'downstream' is in supination while the foot 'upstream' is everted or in talus valgus;

in climbing (fig. 62), the foot 'downstream' must be firmly anchored to the ground perpendicular to the slope, i.e. in a position of pes cavus varus while the foot 'upstream' approaches the ground in maximal flexion and parallel to the slope;

in coming down a slope (fig. 63) the feet must often be inverted so as to secure maximum grip.

Thus, just as the palm of the hand allows prehension by changing its curvature and its orientation in space, the sole of the foot can within limits adapt to the irregularity of the ground so as to ensure optimal contact with it.

234

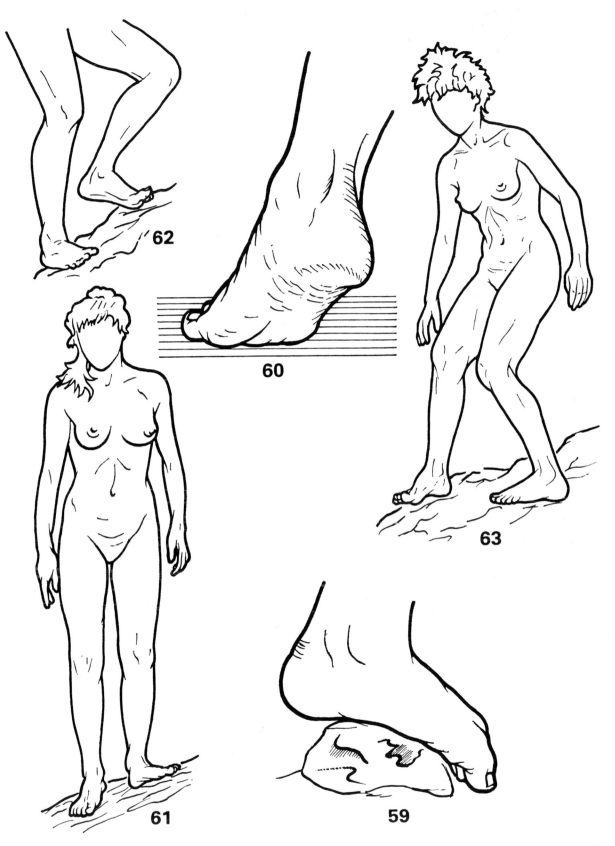

62

60

63

61

59

235

CLAW FOOT (PES CAVUS)

The curvature and orientation of the plantar vault depend upon a very delicate balance of the various muscles concerned. This can be studied with the help of Ombrédanne's model (fig. 64):

the vault is flattened by the weight of the body (white arrow) and by contracture of the muscles attached to the convexity of the vault: the triceps surae (1), the tibialis anterior and the peroneus tertius (2), the extensor digitorum longus and the extensor hallucis longus (3). The last two muscles are effective only if the proximal phalanges are stabilised by the interossei (7);

the vault is 'hollowed' by contracture of the muscles attached to its concave aspect: the tibialis posterior (4), the peroneus longus and brevis (5), the plantar muscles (6) and the flexor digitorum longus (8). It can also be hollowed by a relaxation of the muscles inserted into its convexity. Conversely, relaxation of the muscles in its concavity leads to a flattening of the vault.

Insufficiency or contracture of a single muscle disrupts the overall equilibrium and leads to some deformity. Duchenne de Boulogne states in this connection that it is better to have all the muscles paralysed rather than a single muscle, since then the foot retains a fairly normal shape and position.

There are three types of pes cavus:

1. The 'posterior' type (fig. 65), where the deformity involves the posterior buttress of the plantar vault due to insufficiency of the triceps surae (1). The muscles in the concavity of the arch are inadequately balanced (6) and the sole is hollowed; the ankle flexors (2) tilt the foot in a position of flexion. This leads to the talipes equinus (fig. 66) which is often compounded with a valgus deformity (fig. 67) following contracture of the abductors of the foot (the extensor digitorum longus, the peronei muscles).

2. The 'intermediate' type (fig. 68) is relatively rare and results from contracture of the plantar muscles (6), which can follow the use of shoes with too rigid soles or shortening of the plantar aponeurosis (Ledderhose's disease).

3. The 'anterior' type can be further divided into subgroups which all share an equinus deformity (fig. 69) showing the following two characteristics:

equinus deformity of the forefoot (e) due to lowering of the anterior buttresses of the vault,

a misalignment (d) between the heel and the forefoot, which can be partially reduced when the body weight is being supported.

Depending on the mechanism underlying the condition, the following varieties of the anterior type of pes cavus are described:

contracture of the tibialis posterior (4) and of the peronei longus and brevis (5) causes a lowering of the anterior part of the foot (fig. 70). Contracture of the peronei alone can lead to pes cavus which is then compounded with a valgus deformity, i.e. talipes arcuatus, equinovalgus (fig. 71);

an imbalance of the metatarsophalangeal joints (fig. 72) is a common cause of pes cavus: insufficiency of the interossei (7) tips the balance in favour of the toe extensors (3) and hyperextension of the first phalanx follows. Next the metatarsal heads become lowered (6) and this leads to a lowering of the anterior part of the foot; hence pes cavus;

lowering of the metatarsal heads can also be due (fig. 13) to an insufficiency of the tibialis anterior (2): the extensor digitorum longus (3) attempts to compensate and tilts the proximal phalanges; the plantar muscles (6), now unbalanced, accentuate the curvature of the vault and triceps action provokes a slight equinus deformity. A slight degree of valgus (fig. 74) follows from the inadequately balanced extensor digitorum; hence the condition of talipes arcuatus equino-valgus;

a common cause of clawfoot is the wearing of shoes that are too short, or of high-heeled shoes (fig. 75): the toes hit against the tip of the shoes and are hyperextended (a) so that the metatarsal heads are lowered (b). Under the weight of the body (fig. 76) the foot slides forward down the slope and the heel and toes are approximated. This exaggerates the curvature of the vault.

The diagnosis of claw foot is made easier by studying the footprint (fig. 77). In comparison with the normal footprint (I) the first stage of pes cavus (II) shows a projection on its lateral border (m) and a deepening of the concavity of the medial border (n). The next stage (III) shows a footprint which is divided into two. Finally, in the long-standing cases (IV), these characteristics become associated with the disappearance of the prints of the toes (q) due to a secondary claw-toe deformity.

It must be realised, however, that the footprint typical of the flat foot with an incomplete lateral border can be produced by the talipes planovalgus of children and adolescents. The valgus of the calcaneus and the flattening of the medial arch cause the lateral arch to 'take off' with central loss of contact with the ground. This finding can lead to a misdiagnosis but it is easy to recognize this mimic of the flatfoot footprint as follows:

the toes lie flat on the ground;

when the medial arch is raised or, better still, when the leg is rotated laterally with the foot resting on the ground, the lateral border of the footprint reappears while the medial arch hollows further.

236

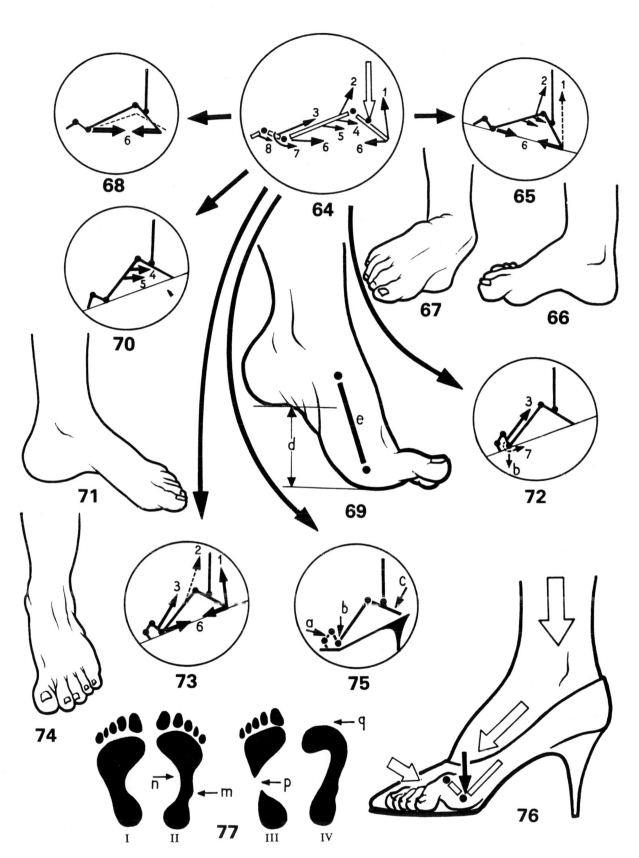

68

64

65

67

66

70

71

69

72

73

75

74

77

76

I II III IV

n m p q

d e a b c

FLAT FOOT (PES PLANUS)

The collapse of the plantar vault is due to *weakness of its natural means of support*, i.e. muscles and ligaments. The ligaments by themselves are capable of maintaining the integrity of the vault for a short period since the footprint of an amputated leg is normal except if the ligaments have been previously cut. In life however, if the muscular support fails, the ligaments become stretched eventually and the vault collapses for good.

The flat foot is therefore due mainly to muscular insufficiency (fig. 78): insufficiency of the tibialis posterior (4) or, more commonly of the **peroneus longus** (5). If the foot is not supporting the body the foot shows a varus deformity (fig. 79) because the peroneus longus is an abductor. On the other hand, when the weight of the body is applied to the foot (fig. 80) the medial arch collapses and a *valgus deformity results*. This valgus is due to two factors:

1. The transverse arch of the foot, normally maintained by the tendon of the peroneus longus (fig. 81), becomes flattened (fig. 82); at the same time the medial arch is lowered: the forefoot (e) rotates medially on its long axis so that the sole of the foot touches the ground over its whole surface and simultaneously the forefoot is displaced (d) laterally.

2. The calcaneus turns on its long axis in the direction of pronation (fig. 83) and tends to lie flat on its medial surface. This degree of valgus, which is visible and can be measured by the angle between the axis of the heel and the Achilles tendon, exceeds the physiological limits (5°) and can attain 20° in certain cases. According to some authors, this valgus deformity is due primarily to a malformation of the articular surfaces of the subtalar joint and an abnormal measure of laxity of the interosseous ligaments; other authors believe these lesions to be secondary.

Whatever the cause, this valgus displaces the centre of stress towards the medial border of the foot and the talar head moves inferiorly and medially. The medial margin of the foot then shows the presence of three more or less distinct *projections* (fig. 82):

the medial malleolus (a), abnormally prominent;

the medial part of the head of the talus (b);

the tubercle of the navicular bone (c).

The tubercle of the navicular represents the apex of the obtuse angle formed by the axes of the posterior and anterior parts of the foot: adduction-pronation of the posterior part is compensated by abduction-supination of the anterior part, so that the curvature of the vault is flattened out. (Hohmann, Boehler, Hauser, Delchef, Soeur).

This complex of deformities has already been described when the static changes of the plantar vault were studied (p. 227, fig. 41). (In this case, they are less marked.) It is a relatively common condition, known as *the painful flat foot or tarsalgia of the young*.

The diagnosis of flat foot is made easier with the use of the **footprint** (fig. 84): in comparison with the normal footprint (I), the concavity of the medial border of the foot is gradually filled out (II and III) until in long-standing cases (IV) the medial border may even become convex.

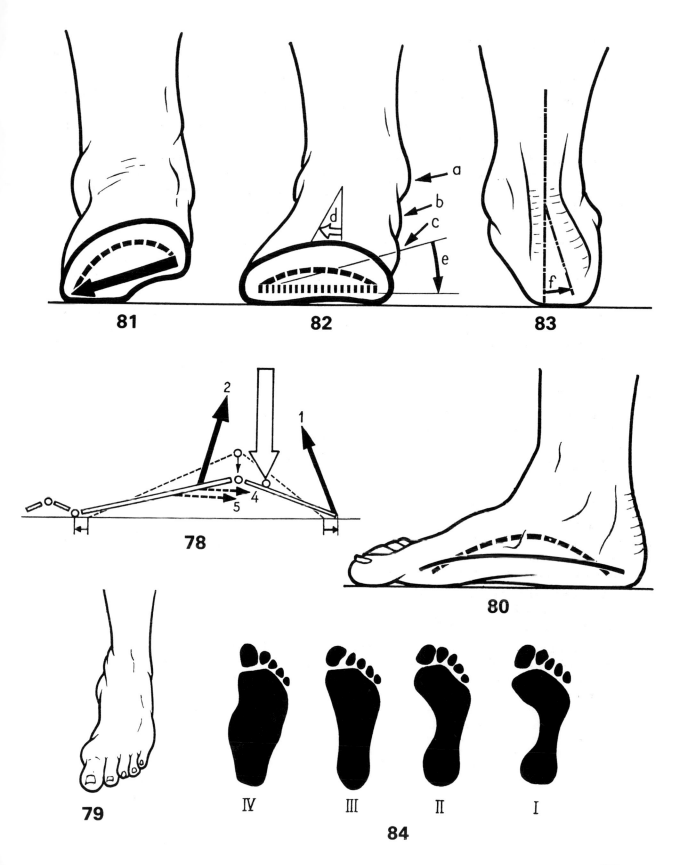

81

82

a
b
c
d
e

83

f

2
1
4
5

78

80

79

IV   III   II   I

84

239

IMBALANCE OF THE ANTERIOR ARCH

In the development of deformities of the plantar vault the balance of the anterior arch can be upset at the level of its **supports** and by changes of its **curvature**.

This imbalance is generally secondary to the anterior type of pes cavus: the equinus deformity of the forefoot enhances the stresses applied to the anterior arch in the following three ways:

1. *The equinus deformity of the anterior part of the foot is symmetrical* (fig. 85), i.e. without any pronation or supination of the foot; the curvature of the arch is preserved. Thus the **two supports become overloaded** and callosities develop under the heads of the first and fifth metatarsals.

2. *The equinus deformity is associated with pronation of the foot* (fig. 86) due to a greater degree of lowering of the medial arch (contracture of the tibialis posterior or of the peroneus longus); as the curvature of the arch is maintained, **the medial support of the arch bears the brunt of the overload** and a callosity develops under the head of the first metatarsal.

3. *The equinus deformity is accompanied by supination of the foot* (fig. 87): the curvature of the arch is maintained and the **lateral support bears the brunt of the overload** (callosity under the head of the fifth metatarsal).

In certain types of anterior pes cavus the curvature of the anterior arch can be altered as follows:

partially flattened or *straightened* (fig. 88): this is the case of the **anterior type of flat foot**; the overload is distributed to all the metatarsal heads (callosity under each head);

completely reversed (fig. 89): this is the **anterior type of round foot**; the overload is borne by the heads of the three middle metatarsals (with corresponding callosities).

Inversion of the anterior arch is due to a claw or hammer deformity of the toes. As we have seen before, this deformity of the toes can result from an imbalance between the interossei and the extensors; very often it results from shoes that are too short or from high heels (which are equivalent to tight shoes): the toes (fig. 90) hit against the front of the shoes and are bent; the head of the first phalanx is pulled down and a callosity appears; the head of the metatarsal is itself lowered (callosity develops) and the arch collapses.

This also occurs readily when pointed shoes are worn on feet of a particular configuration: the **pes anticus** (the Neanderthal foot) which recalls the prehuman foot with the prehensile big toe (fig. 91):

the first metatarsal is short, excessively mobile and set far apart from the second metatarsal (metatarsus varus or adductus) so that the big toe runs obliquely anteriorly and medially;

the second metatarsal is distinctly longer than the others so that it supports the weight during the final phase of the step. It is thus overloaded and pain develops at its base; occasionally fatigue fracture occurs; the fifth metatarsal is widely set laterally (valgus deformity of the fifth metatarsal).

When this widely splayed forefoot is confined within pointed shoes (fig. 92) the big toe is displaced laterally (a). This imbalance soon becomes permanent as a result of shortening of the capsular ligament of the joints, lateral dislocation of the sesamoid bones (c) and of the tendon, the formation of an exostosis (b) and of a callosity on the metatarsal head. This is the pathogenesis of the **hallux valgus**. The big toe displaces the intermediate metatarsals exaggerating their hammer deformity (fig. 93). The fifth toe undergoes the converse deformity: this is the **quintus varus** which further enhances the hammer deformity of the intermediate toes. In this way the anterior arch becomes convex.

The morphologic type of the foot plays an important role in the development of these deformities. In artistic terms there are three types of foot:

the **Greek foot**, as observed in classical Greek statues. The second toe is the longest, followed by the big toe and the third toe, which are nearly of the same length, and then by the fourth and fifth toes. In this type of foot loads achieve their best distribution on the forefoot.

the **Polynesian foot**, or square foot, as seen in Gauguin's paintings, with the toes, at any rate the first three, being of equal length. This foot gives no problems.

the **Egyptian foot**, as seen on statues of the Pharaohs, with the big toe being the longest while the others decrease in length successively. This type of foot is the most prone to problems. The relatively longer big toe is forced laterally in the shoe (hallux valgus) and is unduly stressed during walking, leading to metatarsophalangeal osteoarthritis (hallux rigidus).

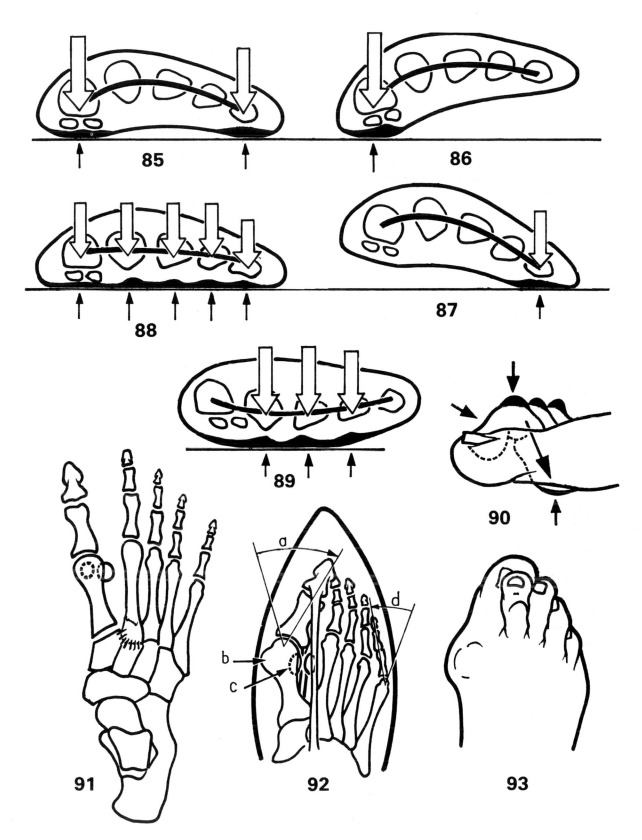

85

86

87

88

89

90

91

92

93

BIBLIOGRAPHY

Barnett CH, Davies DV, Mac Conaill MA 1961 Synovial Joints. Their structure and mechanics. Thomas Ed., Springfield, USA

Barnier L 1950 L'analyse des mouvements. PUF, Paris

Bellugue P 1962 Introduction à l'étude de la forme humaine; anatomie plastique et mécanique. Édition posthume à compte d'Auteur, Paris

Biesalski N, Mayer L 1916—Die physiologische Sehnentransplantation. Springer, Berlin

Bonnel F, Jaeger JH, Mansat C 1984 Les laxités chroniques du genou. 1 vol. Masson, Paris

Dorlot JM, Christel P, Witwoet J, Sedel L 1984 Déplacements des insertions des ligaments croisés durant la flexion du genou normal. Suppl. II, Rev. Chir. Orthop. 70: 50–53

De Doncker E, Kowalski C 1970 Le pied normal et pathologique. Notions d'anatomie, de physiologie et de pathologie des déformations du pied. Extract from Acta Orthopédica Belgica 36: 4–5

Duchenne GBA (De Boulogne), 1867—Physiologie des mouvements. American translation by Kaplan EB 1949 Lippincott, Philadelphia

Fick R 1911 Handbuch des Anatomie und Mechanik g Gelenk Gustav Fischer, Iéna

Fischer O 1907 Kinematik Organischer Gelenke. F. Vierveg & Son, Braunschweig

Frain P, Fontaine C, D'Hondt D Contraintes du genou par dérangement ménisco-ligamentaire. Étude de l'Articulation Condylo-Tibiale Interne. Rev. Chir. Orthop (in press)

Henke W 1863 Handbuch der Anatomie und Mechanik der Gelenke. C.F. Winter, Heidelberg

Kapandji IA 1967 The knee ligaments as determinants of trochleo-condylar profile. Med & Biol. Illustration vol. XVII, p 26–32

Lapidus 1963 Kinesiology and mechanical anatomy of the tarsal joints. Clin Orthop 30: 30–34

Mac Conaill MA 1966 Studies on the anatomy and function of bones and joints. F. Gaynor Evans, New York

Mac Conaill MA 1966 The geometry and algebra of articular kinematics. Bio Med. Eng 1: 205–212

Mac Conaill MA, Basmadjian JV 1969 Muscles and movements; a basis for human kinesiology. Williams & Wilkins Co, Baltimore

Menschik A 1974 Mechanik des Kniegelenkes. Z. Orthop. 112: 481–495

Morton DJ 1935 The human foot. Columbia University Press, New York

Poirier P, Charpy A 1926 Traité d'Anatomie humaine 4th edn. Masson, Paris

Rash PJ, Burke RK 1971 Kinesiology and applied anatomy, 4th edn. Lea Febiger, Philadelphia

Rocher CH, Rigaud A 1964 Fonctions et bilans articulaires. Masson, Paris

Roud A 1918 Mécanique des articulations et des muscles de l'homme. F. Rouge & Co, Lausanne

Rouvière H 1948 Anatomie Humaine descriptive et topographique, 4th edn. Masson, Paris

Segal P, Segal M et al 1983 Le Genou, vol 1. Maloine, Paris.

Steindler A 1955 Kinesiology of the human body. Charles Thomas, Springfield, USA

Strasser H 1917 Lehrbuch der Muskel-und Gelenkmechanik. Springer, Berlin

Testut L 1921 Traité d'anatomie humaine. Doin, Paris

Vandervael F 1956 Analyse des mouvements du corps humain. Maloine, Paris